Contemporary nursing:
Culture, education
and practice

This book is due for return on or before the last date shown below.

Don Gr

Contemporary nursing: Culture, education and practice

by
Liam Clarke

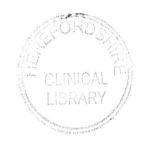

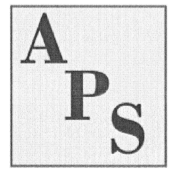

Academic Publishing Services
The Old School, Tollard Royal, Salisbury, Wiltshire, SP5 5PW
www.apspublishing.co.uk

British Library Cataloguing in Publication Data
A catalogue record for this book is available from the British Library

© Academic Publishing Services 2001
ISBN 0 9537234 8 8

Printed in the UK by Selwood Printing Limited, Burgess Hill

Contents

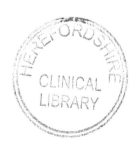

Preface

The topics I have chosen to write about here, all deal in different ways with the themes of power and authority. By whose authority, for instance, should nurses be permitted to prescribe drugs? Should such prescriptive power be seen as a valid indicator of equality between nursing and related professions? How does this square with the radical differences between how nurses and these other professions, notably medicine, are educated? These and many other questions are raised in this book and, hopefully, in a readable way. My playful view has always been that readability and polemic are comfortable bedfellows. As such, please do not enter these pages if anticipating a balanced view. Having said that, there is nothing flippant or superficial here and in some instances, chapter six for instance, the writing was painful and loaded with regret. Initially, I had conceived this book as a psychiatric text, but there are many things here that will be of interest to nurses generally. I should also mention that I have opted for the term psychiatric and not mental health nurse because of the insane formlessness of the latter term. The chapters are designed to be read alone if required and the reader may dip into the book in any sequence of their choosing. However, it will become apparent that the aforementioned themes of power, its acquisition and expression, and authority, its relationship to knowledge and practice, are the twin pillars upon which this book rests.

I want to thank Bill McGowan, trusted colleague, for reading some of the text and making valuable suggestions. The same holds true for my daughter, Martina, whose refreshing 'outsider' comments caused me to alter my thinking. To Johanna Clarke, my wife, whose name could so easily accompany mine on the cover, much thanks. And thanks to Sinéad, who kept me sane and relatively good humoured throughout a crowded schedule.

1
The varieties of nursing

*I*n general, three groups of nurses appear to nervously co-exist with one another. The first group—the positivists—look to the natural sciences to verify their position and are suspicious of theory or practice that departs from positivist, deductive philosophy. It is not that they deny moral standing to patient's experiences, but that they place more emphasis on their clinical status. The second group is more 'person-centred': here, people are seen to possess moral worth, their experiences of the world and their intentionality being viewed as the essence of their psychological status. Their clinical status is secondary.

While it is tempting to think that these two groups might be synonymous with general and psychiatric nurses respectively, this is not so. Clear differences do emerge between general and psychiatric nurses when tested on their attitudes and interests (Caine and Smail, 1981). However, marked differences **within** these groups also emerge, when the profession is viewed from other perspectives, such as management, academia and so on. Within psychiatric nursing, for instance, a debate that reflects the views of both person-centred and positivist nurses has raged for years and continues to do so (Repper, 2000). In general nursing, alternatively, divisions have centred around a minority and a majority. The minority possess a person-centred outlook, but for very different reasons to psychiatric nurses. For the most part their person-centredness has been more to do with acquiring professional autonomy and disowning medical influences. The much larger third group is more pragmatic in its beliefs and practices and has little difficulty working under medical prescription. This group is inclined to be sceptical about academically led pursuits, tending instead to base its working procedures on custom and experience.

So, while differences between nurses range along a continuum, with positivism at one end and person-centeredness at the other, in the case of general versus psychiatric nurses they do so for very different reasons. The arguments within psychiatry seem to be rooted in long standing debates about the nature of mental illness and its treatments. Whereas, in general nursing, the emergence of person-centeredness (linked with holism) seems less a true shift in the nature of belief about illness and more a required bid towards re-creating nursing as a professional entity.

Metaphysics

An indication of the fragility of holism within general nursing is that it frequently lapses into a kind of metaphysics often in association with charismatic leaders. The various 'models of nursing', for instance, are typically stamped by the insights of their founders as they seek to explicate human illness in non-medical and, on occasions, mystical ways.

Albert Ellis (Edwards, 1992) notes that spiritual and transpersonal practitioners tend to have strong beliefs in God-like intuition, higher powers, elevated consciousness and an ability to cure oneself of physical or mental illness. One of the 'leading lights' of this approach is Professor Jean Watson. According to her:

> 'The nurse has a human responsibility to move beyond the patient's immediate specific needs and help the patient reach his or her highest level of growth, maturity and health. Nursing's most important goal is the promotion of self-actualisation'.
>
> (Elliot, 1997)

Fawcett (1993) believes that Watson's theory 'goes beyond the existential-phenomenological approach to, perhaps, a higher level of abstraction and sense of personhood, incorporating concepts of the soul and transcendence' and reaching towards a metaphysical world where 'nothing is random or meaningless' (p218).

Newman's (1993) assumptions—partly drawn from the ideas of Martha Rogers—similarly equate health with an expanding consciousness where 'all opposites are reconciled. Here,' says Newman, 'experiences of all kinds are equal and unconditional; pain as well as pleasure, failure as well as success, ugliness as well as beauty, disease as well as non-disease'. Accordingly, the soul:

> *'moves directly in circular reasonings, where retreats are as important as advances, preferring labyrinth and corners, giving a metaphorical sense to life. Soul is vulnerable and suffers; it is passive and remembers' (p47).*

Perorations on the soul, like these, imply that nurses will discover occupational meaning through their existence, their life experiences. Nursing takes on a mystical, if morally non-directional, ambience and with a presumption that this will bind nurses into some form of universal and expanding consciousness.

The problem with this is that it is hard to see how it connects with practical nursing. There might be room (and psychological need) for metaphysical speculation when, for example, nursing dying patients although, even here, the patient's needs may well be practical, i.e., concerns about offspring, their future well-being, and so on. When one considers the problems of acutely ill people, however, the less relevant metaphysics becomes. The writings of holistic nurses rarely contain any evidence that acutely ill people actively seek the kinds of 'soul comforts', which they seek to provide. Neither is there much testimony from practice nurses (the third category) that patients see their illnesses in metaphorical terms. Yet some (Keighley, 2001) persist in calling for a heightened emphasis on 'the spiritual' in nursing, asserting that the meaning of nursing **is** spirituality.

The meaning of illness

Something which the nursing preoccupation with meaning can do is inculcate in ill people the questionable notion that they may be bringing sickness on themselves. This stems from the Watsonian idea that nothing is random, a belief that can lead to fruitless, punishing searches for sources of guilt and self-recrimination. This kind of soul searching found approval in a post-Thatcherite/Reaganite era, where dependency was viewed as self-inflicted. While holistic philosophers may blanch at the idea of attaching moral blame to people, nevertheless, the implications of their teaching is that disability is part and parcel of who one is and not simply something that 'happens'.

Many nurses have particular difficulties in dealing with questions like these, given their historical inability to connect theoretical issues to broader political and social changes. Compared to other disciplines, there is little nursing discourse on how the profession has developed (or functions) within general political and/or economic frameworks. With a few exceptions (Salvage, 1985; White, 1986; Rafferty, 1996a; 1996b) nursing typically looks to tradition to solve its problems, but the sorry fact is that the nursing tradition has been to react uncritically to untried and even, sometimes, implausible ideas. Possibly nursing lacks the talent to sustain a critical analysis of its role within the wider society. Or the way in which nursing is structured within health systems prevents such an analysis from taking place. Such a critique would, of course, have as its background the broad mass of nurses whose scepticism about most things intellectual remains intact.

Whatever the reason, concepts such as holism (or Nursing Process) are taken up almost as new and different nirvanas and—it should be added—to the despair of the larger, third group, of practice nurses. The absence of a critique is made understandable, however, when you consider that introducing holism was less to do with its philosophical validity and more the fact that its introduction bolstered the claims of an elitist minority in search of 'learned profession' status. For many, their position was already fixed in respect of their dependence on medical perspectives.

The busy ward

I am reluctant to contrast Professor Watson's abstractions with the demands of busy, understaffed wards, inadequate facilities, and the unpredictability of the illness process, but the fact is that nursing is implicated in all of these things. Nurses operate in difficult circumstances, cope with catastrophe, endlessly deal with the mundane as well as the dynamic, and all within the oppressive requirements of shift systems. Historically, the nursing obligation to (and within) the shift system drastically affects the kinds of work that nurses can do. Other disciplines work in treatment centres for limited periods, in respect of particular patients, or with a defined task in mind. It is the time-limited nature of these interventions that makes therapy possible. Alternatively, nurses have, over many years, assumed a responsibility for the intermediary events surrounding the delivery of treatments by the other disciplines. This intermediary role (Towell, 1975) has meant providing 24-hour cover for hospital wards or other treatment units. As such, the idea that nurses could be actively therapeutic across eight-hour shifts seems unlikely. It might be possible, but it is very improbable. What this situation does is to sustain the conditions by which other disciplines provide therapy in a time-limited, objective and supposedly scientific way.

At the same time, a genuine commitment to provide care for sick and confused patients is frequently evident, although increasingly, these days, the care is often at the hands of junior nurses or health care assistants. The struggle to achieve a good level of care is what makes nursing in institutional settings such an unrewarding undertaking. The point being that any account of nursing, which fails to link with these practical aspects necessarily fails. The unworldly nature of spiritual theorising 'flies in the face' of the everyday obligations of nursing: it lacks commonsense to the point of practical uselessness. In cases where nurses do achieve a measure of time management over their role, typically the role becomes something else. For example, in Health Visiting the nursing element is diminished in favour of concerns about public health and illness prevention. In psychiatric practice, some nurses become behavioural therapists where the role shifts again, this time to a specific therapy aimed at particular types of psychological problems.

Something more plausible

We need to look at more plausible nursing theories. Alison Kitson (1993) says that the kind of nurse described by Patricia Benner—author of 'From Novice to Expert' (1984)—is one that makes 'independent judgements on each case within the context of where the care is carried out.' Such a nursing role is said to 'foster healing relationships, decrease alienation, and be a witness to her patient's experience' (Kitson, p41). At face value, this seems a less fanatic espousal of 'other world' mysticism and appears more tied down to 'real world' thinking. For Benner (1984), understanding the patient's experience of illness can be a powerful force for healing even in the absence of other nursing or medical treatments. Benner has been at the forefront in denoting nursing as a 'caring profession', asserting that the human impulse to care is what lies at the heart of treatment and healing. She says that nursing works best when it embraces feminine values, when it does not ape the power values of medicine. The premise: 'If you can't beat them join them' is expressly rejected as constituting a failure to assert the necessity of a caring/feminine role.

There are two things to note about Benner's position. Firstly, the caring that she advocates is, she says, something that occurs at a personal/individual level. Issues relating to collective and/or professional groupings, she does not address. Her insistence that caring is what nursing is about, apart from being a tautology, assumes a level of idealistic practice that is not always found. What happens, for example, if the conditions of caring are deficient (Martin, 1984; Allitt Inquiry, 1994; Stanley *et al*, 1999; Coombes, 2001), and the nurses are unable or unwilling to change them?

The second point is that Benner specifically rejects scientific notions of an independent reality (1984: p216) in favour of 'realities' that are constructed, in part, through language. This language ploy is the most common method used to give parity to nursing perspectives in respect of the medical viewpoint. Its application, however, is frequently inconsistent and frequently not fully worked out. For example, if reality is construed through language, then the manner by which medical language came to influence, even dominate, treatment settings becomes an important focus for study. Yet it is the one focus that nurse theorists ignore, resting their case instead on the supposed 'breakthrough' of **asserting** parity through language.

In the United Kingdom, the conclusions of Professor Celia Davies are not that different from Benner, although she reaches these conclusions via a more solid, sociological route. In her review of feminism and caring, Davies (2000) identifies the medical role as detached and lacking human feeling: while not uncaring, the medical disposition is about 'not being visibly moved, not getting bound up in [the patient's] crises or pain' (p348). Alternatively, nurses engage with patients in a reflective, person-centred way, where care is negotiated and inter-dependant issues are worked through. For Davies, this 'womanly caring' is potentially anxiety-provoking, especially when contrasted with the masculine-driven values of objectivity, distance, and control (i.e., the hallmarks of positivism). Again, one sees that this is an idealised picture, describing what ought rather than what actually is the case. Avoiding the personal worlds of patients, by objectifying one's work through ritual or other distancing manoeuvres, is not unique to the medical profession as anyone familiar with Isabel Menzies' (1960) paper 'Social Systems as a Defence against Anxiety' knows. All told, there is insufficient evidence to conclusively link caring and gender (Handford, 1994) and it is not too improbable that in equally problematic settings females may be just as 'distant' as males. That said, nurses generally have become less procedural and more interpersonal in their work, although obtaining a true picture is difficult given the aspirational cum inspirational statements of the minority, which act to camouflage the activities of the majority.

The dilemma seems to be that nurses either emulate what Davies calls the 'hero professional' role, operating essentially 'on the outside' and swooping down when needed to provide curative therapy, or else to follow a less delineated role, one of carer/advocate, perhaps, where the demarcation between carer and cared-for is more diffuse. While neither of these writers, Benner or Davies, addresses the practice concerns of the majority of nurses, they do advance matters beyond the spiritual meandering of writers like Watson.

Novices and experts

In her book 'From Novice to Expert', Benner described a caring rhetoric firmly linked to events within patient settings, but exhibiting little of the religious veneer of some of her contemporaries. The book also won many adherents because of the importance it then rightly placed on gender issues. Davies, an interesting British voice in an area dominated by American writing, added that future changes will require discussions not only about gender, but about race and class as well. On the question of class, for example, the majority of nurses, identified here as pragmatic in their views, come from predominantly social classes IV and V. Almost the whole of this group belong to general nursing and, notwithstanding recent innovations in nurse education, have persistently rejected concepts of nursing as theory led. Specifically, these nurses objected to the introduction into their curricula of socio-political (including feminist) dimensions at the expense of anatomy and physiology, and pathology-based teaching. It is this chasm between a largely pragmatic majority and over-idealised schemes, such as Benner's, that constitutes a major problem in nursing. Because, in addition to ignoring the contextual constrains already outlined, what the 'nurse philosophers' also avoid are such things as the prescriptive role of doctors, the reality of pathology-based illness, the economics of health care provision, and the fundamental medical needs of patients: in effect, the very things that the broad mass of nurses identify with.

Other voices

It is against this background of widespread practice that we need to evaluate not just the proselytising of spirituality nurses, but the more modified positions of Benner and Davies as well. For instance, how do writers, such as Benner and

Watson, connect with the broader stream of humanistic writers, like Abraham Maslow (1987) or Carl Rogers (1978) whose influence on nursing has been far reaching. Indeed, it is Rogers who has bequeathed to modern nursing its language and overall veneer of person-centred and holistic practice. Not so, says British nurse Alison Kitson (1993), the nurses' use of humanistic principles differs from Rogers (and the counselling psychology to which he gave rise) and the difference, says Kitson:

> 'Lies in the way the nurse chooses to use them; in the therapeutic paradigm a number of rules and principles would come into play, while in the ethical paradigm the nurse responds to the patient as a person and establishes a caring relationship based on mutual realisation. While the therapeutic caring relationship may claim the same features, again the distinction is in relation to how the nurse decides what to do, how engaged she becomes and how authentic her communications with the other person' (p41).

Now, I am puzzled as to how this differs from Maslow or Rogers. Indeed, Rogerians would probably regard as cheek, the suggestion that nurses bring authenticity to encounters. Which is not to say that they do not. It's just that their humanism hardly characterises what nursing is unless you accept that it is somehow synonymous with counselling. Such comparisons are meaningless, however, and the person-centred group seems not to have moved nursing beyond membership of a counselling fraternity whose distinguishing characteristics are just as hard to define as their own.

All in all, the transpersonalism of writers like Watson and Fawcett has little to offer nurses whose problem is to cope with people in medical need. Its modification by people, like Davies and Benner, provides a more credible basis upon which to continue discussion, but still does not advance us very far. The person-centred and holistic attitude is retained, even if a more independent nursing role is asserted, on the grounds of their gender-inherited status as befrienders and advocates. Nevertheless, Benner and Davis have raised points of considerable importance. Is it the case, for instance, that a male dominated medical profession is distanced and objective because it is male? Or does medical practice **require** objectivity and distance if it is to be safe and efficient? Upon what, exactly, is the assumption that male doctors lack feeling or respect for persons—a common currency amongst nurses—based? And, lastly, granted that nurses do implement caring strategies that reflect holistic and subjective concerns, do these add significantly to the medical diagnoses and treatments, which must necessarily dominate hospitals and clinics?

Common ground

Outside of clinical nursing—which is medical by nature—there cannot, in my view, be a nursing knowledge since the practise-base of nursing lies within clinical settings and is always closely associated with medical practice. I use the term medical setting in its widest possible sense. For example, NHS Direct (1997), the 'first aid' telephone system manned by nurses, is a service staffed by 'specially trained' (i.e. medically trained) nurses. Within such settings, nurses could not act pursuant to a non-medical expertise: likewise, in a hospital, they could not act from holistic considerations if such actions violated medical prescriptions.

Of course, there may be much to nursing that does not violate medical practice, but actually complements it. The care of the dying is one such area, as is also caring for people with chronic impairments. In such cases, person-centred nurses may not be concerned with questions of epistemology, choosing instead to construct their role on the basis of personal encounters with patients. Not surprisingly, some nurse theorists have tried to create forms of 'knowing' on the basis of such encounters, arguing that nurses develop insights into patient's problems precisely from their experience of being with them. Knowledge emerges through verbal interchanges with 'significant others' and is sometimes called narrative or discourse knowledge. Bruni (1991) challenges the standing of this new knowledge in terms of how it relates to medicine. According to Bruni, such discourse-knowledge 'does not challenge the existing occupational hierarchy' (p174) other than in non-clinical settings, such as educational institutes and/or organisations dedicated to preventative and public health care. In other words, most debates that examine power sources between doctors and nurses occur outside clinical settings and especially if debate touches on theoretical issues. Interestingly, Davies (2000) recalls that her attempts to discuss nursing from the vantage point of feminism were met with scepticism by nursing colleagues.

Illness

The occurrence of illness is basic to this discussion. The positivist tradition derives its power from knowledge of pathology and illness and the curative powers of a scientifically informed medical practice. Holistic or person-centred approaches view illness as but an inter-related element in the general life of the person. For them, illness needs to be understood, not only in terms of its pathology, but also in how it is experienced by patients and the role of that experience [for good or ill] on the development of their illness. A problem with this position is that, as holism came to be distilled through one nursing model after another, it gave rise to stock responses to patients and, often, so as to reflect the model being used, nurses became concerned about areas of questionable relevance to their patient's illnesses, for example aspects of their sexuality and personal relationships. Added to which, adopting holism led nurses into transpersonal considerations of why patients had become ill to begin with. As well as quasi-moral attempts to blame illnesses on certain life-styles, there also occurred attempts to re-define physical illness in metaphorical terms.

The problem with playing down illness is that it belittles what matters to patients **at the time of their illness**: explanations which define 'illness as something else' (Fox, 1993), something whose meaning derives from abstractions, only results in detached, formulaic responses to living pain where, in effect, the 'something else' is preferred to the illness. 'Why', asks Susan Sontag (1983), 'can't illness just be illness?' Why indeed. Except that, from a psychiatric perspective, concepts of illness are not so easily dealt with. And, as I have shown, neither can illness be accepted in a straightforward way by holistic practitioners: they are obliged to follow their theory through by examining the significance of illness from a variety of angles. Most of this theorising is, of course, anathema to the positivist group and to whom I now turn.

The positivists

The most vociferous of the positivists come from psychiatric nursing. In the first place, they differ from person-centred nurses in that they see nursing's future as dependent on a close liaison with medicine or clinical psychology. At times, their desire to embrace treatment rather than nursing modalities almost borders on caricature. In terms of mimicking medicine, for example, the current vogue is to prescribe as well as administer medicines, to develop so-called 'nursing diagnoses' and to seek appointments, not as nursing consultants, but as consultant nurses. Most importantly, positivist nurses have sought to define what they do as therapy and to look for scientific explanations in support of their position. While the place of relationships in health care is not denied, they share in the (nowadays frenetic) conviction that physical science explanations are the 'bottom line' in human knowledge and that other forms of 'knowledge', while interesting, are of lesser importance.

Unfortunately, the positivists, as well as the person-centred-group, fail to show how nursing can achieve even a modest occupational autonomy. What they cannot see is that, by adopting medical or psychological interventions, they leave nurses vulnerable to accusations that they are merely second-level or substitute therapists. Yet, notwithstanding this, the positivist case is pressed hard so as to 'lift' nursing from the fuzzy world of second rate philosophising and general ineffectiveness, which they see as the hallmark of person-centred groups.

For the positivists, the way forward is empiricism, in the sense of quantitative measurement, randomised controlled trials, and 'collaborative research' with medicine and psychology. These positivist nurses can be aggressive, combining as they do a scientistic veneer with a 'not suffer fools gladly' dimension added on. What seems lacking in this group is any appreciation that the nursing obligation might be to protect patients from the excesses of scientific applications, to be 'on the outside' of the experimenters, questioning the nature and/or effect of their actions on patients. Professor of Nursing, Philip Barker (Personal communications), comments that:

> *'most nurses accept that they either choose to follow their own star or follow the piper. I do not believe that we could make any progress in the field were there not a sufficient number of non-conformists who refuse to accept local custom and practice harmful to the people in our care'.*

Positivist nurses would hardly accept that they harm people: yet given that another profession already 'owns' the medical knowledge-base, they cannot reasonably expect to achieve autonomy along medical lines. Neither can they lay claim to psychological techniques, such as cognitive-behaviour therapy, without forfeiting the claim to a separate identity.

Of course, this craving for a different identity is about effectiveness and accountability, about evidence and professional respectability: that is, nursing as a rational, communicable and accessible activity. Yet it seems unnatural to exchange, for a measure of therapeutic power, all traces of what might be distinctive about practical nursing. Rather should nurses seek to give shape and purpose to what might be special about what they do. The positivists have set their face against such an enterprise and, from a philosophical viewpoint, probably see such undertakings as redundant. It is true that, in nursing, the quality of philosophising, from an analytic perspective, has not been of the first order. But this does not detract from the moral or professional importance of nurses examining their work and its place in society. Untangling the problems of nursing is, at least, a lively activity, intellectually candid and open to critique.

The third group examined

The third group comprises the broad mass of practising nurses who inhabit the hospitals, treatment centres and community settings that comprise the practice area. The main characteristic of these nurses is their pragmatic acceptance of the basic tenets of medical practice. They might occasionally caution against a too enthusiastic application of medical treatments, but do not challenge the authority of medicine, or their alliance with it in practical terms. Rarely, for example, do nurses and doctors differ in respect of how patients are treated. Inside psychiatric and general nursing practice, the established convention is for nurses to influence medical decisions informally, even surreptitiously, a process brilliantly captured by Leonard Stein (1978) in his paper 'The doctor-nurse game'.

There is, for example, only one recorded case of psychiatric nurses objecting to the use of electric treatment in principle (Bailey, 1983). Two students complained about what they saw as a barbaric treatment and, on ethical grounds, refused to take part. They were dismissed from their posts. It is unlikely that their dismissal prohibited further objections since, actually, most psychiatric nurses favour this treatment. Why should nurses object to something that has stood the test of time and is believed, by most practitioners, to be an effective treatment? For many nurses the 'evidence of their eyes' is an important guardian of truth, so that if something has been seen to work consistently, then it acquires occupational currency. Such nurses are generally unwilling to philosophise about their work and, as we have seen, one particular criticism was the way in which Project 2000 courses pushed theory at the expense of practice. A constant surprise to these nurses is how the person-centred minority behave as if the majority (and its concerns) were of little value. For over 30 years, nurses have been subjected to a 'nursing knowledge' campaign, which has alienated them as well as creating an ever-widening theory-practice gap. Although the minority persist in asserting the 'reality' of patient-centeredness (Fulford, 1996), according to Roger Higgs (1996), it may hardly figure as part of the scenery at all. It is a kind of professional mirage, extraordinarily attractive in the distance and something devoutly to be wished, but, in fact, of little or no utility.

The medical ascendancy

The uncomfortable truth is, that outside of psychiatry, no group has seriously challenged medical dominance, whether in hospital or other treatment settings: all told, even psychiatric dissidents have been few and far between. In general medicine, they are fewer still and, for all of the ostentatious claims of nursing philosophers, it is embarrassingly the case that most practising nurses accept medical jurisdiction. Appearances can be deceiving though, and social interactions between nursing and medical teams often **suggest** fundamental changes in roles and responsibilities. Because many contemporary occupational groups operate along superficially egalitarian lines—first names being the norm, for example—such collegiality does not necessarily mean an abrogation of medical responsibility. That the nurse is no longer 'the doctor's handmaiden' represents a change in the social mores of medical settings. It does not represent an expansion of nursing or a contraction of medical responsibilities.

May (1993) states that doctors exercise authority by virtue of the fact that hospitals are treatment centres: one might add that they are also inhabited by sick people. Within such centres, doctors derive their authority by the nature of their training. The nursing critique of this authority is derived from holism, as well as a new-found preoccupation with health, the latter a strange claim when you consider that most nurses continue to work in hospitals. Unsurprisingly, these 'healthists' avoid phrases like 'treatment centre' or 'hospital'. For example, in a recent debate (see Garbett, 1996) Joyce Zerwekh of the Seattle University Nursing School stated that it was vital to eradicate the prejudice that:

> 'nursing is just common sense; that within a **health care system** [my highlight] peoples' true needs are medical and other types of care are frivolous' (pp42–3).

Of course, within such 'systems' people's medical needs may be relative to other things. For most people though, I submit that it is the occurrence of illness—real or imagined—which forces them to seek help and that, in most instances, they will look to the medical profession for that help. If the help is embodied, in the first instance, by an ancillary (paramedic) or nursing team, the point is that what these teams 'deliver' will be on 'licence' from a medical authority. Independent medical judgements made by nurses, usually follow a protocol or pre-arranged formula that has been set up through medical agreement. If nurses evolve separate systems of non-medical interventions, these may possess authority, but only if they acquire parity with medical judgements. Scott (1998) argues that any nursing authority, which is not based on clinical expertise—and nursing is a practice-based profession—is flawed. This has the effect of moving the discussion away from abstract model building (and mysticism) and towards a concern with the nature of knowledge and/or experience. But what can nurses' clinical experience be if not medical in nature? What nurses claim to know about the caring dimension of their work is rarely discussed in clinical terms: by definition, the person-centred literature actually disavows expertise. Alternatively, the positivist group celebrate expertise, but it is an expertise skilfully appropriated from outside nursing. That they seem well satisfied with themselves does not solve the question of what it is that nurses do: what makes them qualitatively different to other disciplines.

No further on

All in all, we are no further on in finding out what a nursing authority would look like. Clearly, the person-centred nurses have the (quasi religious) authority of their 'calling', although many would reject the 'calling' tag and its religious connotation. It is an authority of sorts, but a long way from an authority derived from clinical expertise. The latter is an improvement on definitions based on 'calling', but its drawback is that it re-aligns nursing with medicine and its accompanying distance and objectivity. That said, it appears to be where most nurses 'are at', which is working side-by-side with medics and with little or no difficulty in doing that.

Commenting on how medical practice came to colonise hospitals, Rafferty (1996a) suggests that, from early on, nurses were co-opted into this system in a secondary and possibly subservient role. Had nursing developed from a domiciliary base, she says, it would today possess more autonomy and professional standing. Rafferty's discussion is largely to do with general nursing, but is helped by looking at how psychiatric nursing had developed in the community. From the early 1950s, a time of upheaval in psychiatric practice, psychiatric nurses had begun to re-direct their interests towards community psychiatry. However, this rarely extended beyond questions of resourcing and caseload management. With hindsight, much could have been expected from psychiatric nurses had they not persisted in their close alignment with the medical profession. Indeed, throughout the psychiatric radicalism of the 1960s and 1970s, community psychiatric nurses at no time questioned conventional psychiatric theory, or their role in implementing it. Ironically, while happy to ignore so-called 'anti-psychiatry', some would later seize upon the humanistic 'philosophies', adopting a counselling perspective with consummate ease. These perspectives would, however, dissipate with the closure of mental hospitals and the consequent political demands that nurses once more address the needs of psychotic patients. Rafferty's assumptions about 'what might have been' for general nursing are hardly born out by the psychiatric nursing experience. In general, it seems as if the geography of practice (see *Chapter 9*) has little influence on how a profession allied to medicine develops.

By whose authority?

In the end, the question is by whose authority do nurses act towards patients? If it is a nursing authority, can it be defined? Is its nature uniform and unambiguous? Or are there as many authorities as there are nursing factions? The medical profession, by contrast, has many specialties, but is united by its commitment to physical sciences as its theoretical base. This is not true for nurses. Indeed, it may be an absence of authority that has allowed nurses to skirt around these issues for so long, chopping and changing from one model to another and rarely affecting a knowledge or ethical standpoint acceptable to most of its members.

Approaching the question differently, which knowledge would patients be prepared to accept; whose knowledge would they trust? A lot might depend on what they thought was the matter with them. If they were beyond medical help, then they might seek solace from nurses. If acutely ill, on the other hand, while some might happily consult nurses about their ailments, it would not be because of what nursing could do for the illness per se. In those cases where nurses **are** enabled to 'treat' an illness, this is done under medical supervision and following some medical training.

So, where does this leave us? On the one hand, nursing is over-romanticised, by Professor Watson and others, into something ethereal and probably impractical in most circumstances. The person-centred approach, defined as a caring, counselling disposition, is no less vague, yet curiously pervasive in contemporary western society. It is this group that has been behind recent developments in nurse education. These educational gains have been short-lived, however, and already the Project 2000 Syllabus is capitulating to the practical demands of the majority of nurses; for example, the re-emergence of 'practical rooms' in nursing institutes, although nowadays, they are normally called 'skills laboratories'.

The positivists are on safer ground: buttressed by new discoveries in molecular sciences, they will continue to affirm their commitment to medical orthodoxy. However, they have foresworn any chance of working out whatever it is nursing might be, having pretty much concluded that nothing is to be gained by intellectual or moral soul searching.

Conclusion

The practical problems of nursing are embodied within the pragmatic majority who deliver practical care under medical jurisdiction. Happy to steer clear of theoretical models, they combine medical know-how and all-round regard for their patients into an imprecise, but comprehensive 'basic nursing care'. Freed from the constraints of academia, the pragmatic nurse advocates on behalf of patients and articulates their views and concerns. When medicine has nothing to offer patients, nurses still care for them and it is this impetus that distinguishes nursing and gives it meaning. This stance is a far cry from the transpersonal and academic pretensions affirmed by a minority. The latter, while idealistic, have contributed significantly to debates about the 'professionalising' of nursing. The positivists share the professional aspirations of the transpersonalists, but they question their inability to account for nursing interventions in a factual way.

A problem for nursing is how to forge the kinds of conditions that would allow these three groups to co-exist, to begin to influence each other: not in any 'conversion' sense, but more in terms of accepting the validity of their different contributions. What I am suggesting resembles Plato's ideal state in 'The Republic' (Penguin Edition, 1955). Here, the workers perform most of the basic tasks and are happy to do so. Above them are the rulers (or philosopher kings) who are specially selected and groomed to rule by rational (evidenced-based) thought and action. Both parties are essentially contented with their built-in inequality. Lastly, there is an administrative group that directs and audits the performance of the workers while interpreting the theories and directives of the ruling elite.

Plato did not expect that his system could come about overnight: in many ways it was an aspiration. It provided for order, but also for well managed innovation and it recognised the unequal roles that different groups have within society. He believed that it was important for the rulers to work on behalf of the others (a crucial element) and he recognised that many would not **want** the obligations that go with ruling. That being the case, they must not seek the kinds of rewards, which go to the ruling classes. Equals must be treated equally of course, but unequals cannot be. This principle is attributed to Aristotle and forms the basis of all theories of distributive

2
Nurse education today

A fter a lengthy apprenticeship, nurse education has now reached an impasse. It is having to rediscover that which it thought it had left behind, as a pre-requisite to the next stages in its development. I shall argue that the Project 2000 innovation, which has governed nurse education in Britain this last fifteen years, was ill conceived, ill thought out—especially its common foundation elements—and completely inappropriate as a preparation for nursing practice. It is my view that an essential characteristic of this misconception was a failure to recognise that the majority of practising nurses did not (and do not) see its relevance in respect of their everyday work. In addition, I will examine the political pressures which came into play following the implementation of Project 2000 and relate these to issues of gender.

The discussion is placed within debates about educational change generally; for example, the implications for nursing were it to withdraw from higher education. Finally, the difficult position of psychiatric nurses within Project 2000 will be reviewed, particularly their loss of curriculum control and the struggle to retain autonomy within an educational framework that pays lip service to, but does not actually appreciate, the different kinds of work that psychiatric nurses do.

Central dilemma

The central dilemma facing nurse education stems from the inception of Project 2000—a supposedly revolutionary development that challenged many of the ways in which nursing was traditionally viewed. Prior to this development, nurses were trained, not educated, and this is a distinction that is not as subtle as might first appear. Indeed, it is not obviously clear how the practical application of nursing—particularly medical/surgical nursing—was to benefit from its new-found association with academia.

The dilemma is two faced. To begin with, there is no evidence that practice based nurses wanted Project 2000 and, as a close analysis by John Humphreys (1996) shows, given half a chance, many would have spurned it. Equally, there is now growing evidence (Le Var, 1997a; 1997b; Hart, 1994) that Project 2000 was championed by a coterie of London-based nurses occupying influential positions both in the government and other agencies, principally the Royal College of Nursing. This dichotomy between an elitist group whose priorities were to do with academia and a larger, practical, workforce was to be the constant destabilising factor for Project 2000 and its implementation.

Like other groups, nursing has had to grapple with the factors that divide and sub-divide its ranks; for example, the vexed problem of how to reconcile a burgeoning, if scrappy, knowledge base with concerns about nursing as a 'bedside activity'. Over the years various attempts have been made to lure and keep nurses 'by the bedside'. For example, the 1974 Halsbury pay award (Rivett, 1998) shortened the differentials between salaries at different levels of the nursing hierarchy, but while these differentials remained static for service staff, they did not prevent the inexorable rise of an (extremely influential) academic clique. This led, ultimately, to a separation of practice from education and the absorption of nurse education into the university system.

These movements took place against a background of radical expansion of higher education generally (Walden, 1996) and, on reflection, it seems hard to see how nurses could have remained outside this expansion. For those who believed that putting a practice-based occupation within the university system was implausible, nursing could look to medicine as an example of a university based enterprise successfully linked to hospital practice. The problem for nurses was that it possessed nothing like the unity of theory and practice forged by medicine over two hundred years. In fact, nursing practice was closely linked to **medical** theory, lacking its own, and this, of course, remains a sticking point. With the advent of Project

2000, however, even this link was weakened. Whereas the older nurse training schools had formed an integral part of the preparation of nurses—partly by their proximity to hospitals—the Project 2000 courses necessitated the movement of students on to the campuses of the newer universities. Equally, there occurred a perceptible playing down of the practical skills of nursing. For instance, clinical teachers (whose role directly related to student's acquisition of practical, ward-based, skills) were phased out and nurse teachers were now required to equip themselves (forthwith) with university degrees, their title now altered to lecturer, and the moral and pastoral responsibilities of the tutor role now abandoned. In place of practical skills, a concern with holistic person-centred care emerged, partly as a substitute for medical theory and partly as an element of budding professionalism.

Digging deeper

Far more was afoot than the re-organisation of nurse training, its integration into higher education, or parity with other education programmes. For the elitists, questions quickly began to address the very nature of nursing, its relationship to medicine, hospitals, and society at large. In a sense, Project 2000 would be the vehicle for a new and 'much improved' profession, one no longer dependent on medicine, but, instead, an autonomous body with its own unique approach to patient care. This uniqueness factor, however, has been the 'new' profession's biggest stumbling block.

The founders of Project 2000, for example, immediately faced the difficulty of how to account for differences between medicine and nursing in knowledge terms. While the idea of a separation between nursing and medicine might seem far-fetched, Project 2000, nevertheless, aimed to turn out preventative, community-based practitioners. The implication was that hospital-based medical-surgical practice was being downgraded. In effect, nurses were attempting to redefine their responsibilities—the nature of their profession—by opting for holism as a working (and philosophical) framework, a framework in which person-centred 'caring' would occupy centre stage. Practical holism would not be a difficulty since it could be construed as synonymous with good multidisciplinary care—something nurses were already used to—and which did not extend to challenging medical priorities. Philosophical holism, on the other hand, carried implications, in respect of the nature of illness, that much more was involved than the physical facts of the case and that nurses might be best placed to minister to patients over and above whatever was medically prescribed.

Holism

The author has dealt with the relationship of nursing to holism elsewhere (Clarke 1999a). For now, it is enough to say that those who espouse holism seem to have forgotten that nursing is a practice-based occupation, whose historical identity emerged over centuries of caring for the sick. Even today, (Firby, 1990) would-be nurses look to hospitals as the proper context for what they imagine nursing to be; there is no evidence that aspiring nurses seek the preventative, healthist or holistic forms of education advocated by Project 2000 enthusiasts.

If holism constitutes the software of the new nurse education, then the common foundation programme (CFP) is its hardware. The role of the CFP within the overall framework is complex, devious, and profoundly mistaken. The CFP derived from an assumption that common elements are relevant to all forms of nursing: this is interesting because it suggests that these common elements can be defined. Without these common foundation elements, nursing would veer off into different interests, interests that might require different definitions: for example, psychiatric nurses would be faced with the difficulty of explaining their participation in compulsory treatments of certified patients. The rhetorical and conceptual (albeit superficial) attractiveness of the CFP headed off these qualitative differences between the branches of nursing and, for a while, it appeared to work.

Of course **some** elements are common to the different divisions of nursing. Few nurses, for example, would deny an obligation to respect the autonomy of their patients or to act with justice towards them. These qualities, however, are available to, or are a part of, humanity as a whole: they are hardly definitive of nursing and their reconstitution within CFPs brought nothing new into nursing. What was distinct about the different branches of nursing, remained.

Not the least of what distinguishes these different branches is the nature of physical as opposed to mental illness. For instance, the fact that significant numbers of mentally ill people are **compelled** to accept treatment fundamentally differentiates mental nurses from their general counterparts. Psychiatric nurses are deeply involved in the use of compulsion—in some legally defined instances they instigate it—and have historically combined a custodial, as well as caring role. Morrall (1998) goes as far as describing this custodial (he calls it policing) role as the central nursing function. While that is debatable, custodialism is, nevertheless, an indispensable element in any discussion about the meaning of psychiatric nursing. Whatever that meaning might be, discussions that helped to illuminate this, and other issues, were severely hampered by the implementing of CFPs and the way in which these programmes quickly came to reflect the concerns and anxieties of general (now called adult) nurses. Not that these concerns were clear-cut. Indeed, the CFP was to become a battlefield upon which the ambitions of those who favoured Project 2000 fell foul of the hopes and expectations of successive student intakes. What the founders of Project 2000 failed to note was that, while the academic expectations of the new courses were strengthened, the student intakes remained constant. In other words, the educationalists continued to 'fish in the same pond' for candidates, while assuming that their notions of what nursing ought to be had somehow entered the consciousness of nursing applicants. Unsurprisingly, the latter would be stunned at what lay in store for them. In fact, the oceans of sociological, psychological, and nursing theory (the latter seen as a special irritant) foisted on CFP students would alienate many of them—especially the general nursing students—whose perceptions of nursing continued to revolve around medicine.

What happens next?

So what is the present position? We have a university-based nursing education, reflecting the ambitions of an upwardly mobile group who seem convinced that, in person-centred holism, they have stumbled upon a viable alternative to medical knowledge. The modularised courses that operationalise these ideas are being delivered to increasingly disgruntled students who appear at odds with these underlying beliefs, and who yearn, instead, for a practice-based training connected to the needs of sick people.

These worries became public knowledge towards the close of the last millennium, when the then Secretary of State for Health, Frank Dobson, began to rail against Project 2000. Its academic 'pretensions' and lack of practical relevance were giving him cause for concern and he began to demand change. Mr Dobson's concerns were immediately refuted by 'spokespersons for the profession', particularly the Royal College of Nursing. These refutations were adept at ignoring findings from research that went some way towards substantiating Dobson's position. In essence, these findings (Robinson, 1991; Macleod Clark *et al*, 1996) identified the CFP as **the** major headache, together with the over-dominance of general nursing concerns and the consequent playing down of the interests of psychiatric students. Much was also made of the lack of contact with practical issues, coupled with what was seen as an undue stress on 'academia'. Significantly, while these findings might ordinarily have been seen as impediments to the continuation of these courses, the researchers concerned, some of whom were involved in Project 2000 courses, were inclined to treat these findings as 'teething problems'. In fact, they were in the nature of a 'running sore' needing urgent attention.

However, in these matters, it is not in the nature of things to move quickly or radically: also, acknowledging failure at this point would have meant, for many, a loss of face. In addition, because the Project 2000 venture was relatively new, it was anticipated by many that a bit of tinkering would solve its problems. Yet the idea that **some** change was inevitable took hold and there then followed a series of 'improvements' that are, in fact, ongoing. The CFP was shortened by six months to one year with the remaining two thirds of each course catering to the specific requirements of each branch, as well as, at last, attempting to link theoretical issues to practical outcomes. This latter point is crucial and its implications have, even yet, to be recognised. For if, from here on, nurse educational programmes are to be practice-led rather than theory-led (and this seems now to be the case) at what price to the place of nurse education within the university system? While universities have had to face the realities of corporate (economic) survival, thus leading them to cut back on, for instance, philosophy departments, in general they would still give precedence to ideas over practice. Historically, as a reading of the Robbins Committee on Higher Education (1963) will show, it was the nursing refusal to give priority to ideas that kept it excluded from higher education. That nursing will remain within higher education seems certain, since it provides much needed income for the universities involved. That nursing **ought** to remain within university systems is another matter. What will happen, ultimately, I suppose, is that nurse education will revert to a training, which will equip nurses to work alongside medical teams in treatment settings. The problem is how to incorporate the aspirations of the minority who remain committed to the notion of an independent nursing profession. Before dealing with this, I propose to dwell, briefly, on the issue of gender.

The slight diversion

Having taught student nurses for over 20 years, my impression is that the majority of them (who are females) care little about 'the women's movement', feminism, or female issues generally. Although a small number of psychiatric nurses do appear to have concerns about these issues, in general nursing you would be hard put to detect much interest in women's issues at all.

And yet, the recent history of nursing can be seen as an emergent culture of autonomy, a series of attempts at forging an independent nursing identity—while shedding the time-worn handmaiden label—mirroring, to some extent, the ascendant role of women generally. I mention this because gender is an excellent barometer of the tensions I have described operating within the CFP and particularly the way in which it fosters division and dissent. Once again, the picture is of a minority who express strong views about, for example, the socio-political-feminine status of nurses (Halford, 1997), but with the majority remaining largely uninvolved. It is on this basis (of ambivalence) that 'the profession' works its way through its problems. At the same time, practising nurses seem barely aware of ethical or professional difficulties between themselves and the medical profession on grounds of gender. One might have anticipated, for instance, that recent controversies in the practice of gynaecology—the area of most complaint about medical negligence—would have elicited a collective ethical response from nurses. This has not happened. Midwifery, however, has evolved a radical stance towards obstetrical procedures and, consequently, midwives are keen to maintain a separate identity from nursing.

Of course, the rules by which professions relate to each other have changed in line with changing mores about social groups generally. Nurses, today, would rightly resent attempts to treat them as second class. They would expect doctors to respect their nursing role, as well as their essential place within treatment teams. That being the case, the 'nurse as handmaiden' model is truly dead. That said, the kind of mutual respect that occupational groups now (rightly) show each other does not impinge on the powers and obligations of each group. What concerns us here, however, is the question of who delivers 'basic nursing' care and whether this can be split from the kind of nursing that draws its authority from the universities and now sees itself in a therapeutic role. If so, then presumably a return to some form of training might be more sensible for the majority who appear to lack sympathy for nursing as a theoretical enterprise.

Let us look at this in more detail. What, for instance, should the role of higher education be in respect of practice-based professions? If nursing is practice based, then should membership come exclusively through higher education programmes, or should such programmes be optional? Further, how does an academic education affect the occupational conditions of post qualification practice: in other words, are nurses adequately prepared? Also, in comparison with other occupations, and educational change generally, what might the repercussions be if nurse education was re-graded to its previous training status? Lastly, there is the question of political resistance to the 'educating up' of gender-biased professions: would Secretary of State Dobson's concerns (and those of others) have been expressed in quite the same way, and with the same vigour, if nursing was not a mainly female occupation?

University standard

An important issue is whether educating nurses requires courses to be set at university standard. However, to do justice to this question, we need firstly to examine whether contemporary degrees represent the standard that pertained when university degrees were a rarer commodity. We now have over 1.7 million people in the university system—not counting nurses—as opposed to about 217 000 in 1965 (Walden, 1996). These figures imply that the meaning of what nowadays counts as a university career is different from before. No longer is the BA Degree the prerogative of a small number of predominantly middle-class adolescents graduating from Eng. Lit or Geography departments. The post-Thatcherite campus is not the rarefied milieu it used to be. For one thing, being more crowded, its facilities are stretched beyond what could have been comprehended even 20 years ago. The resulting desire to generate income has resulted in the welcome mat being put down for what used to be regarded as vocational courses and with entrance criteria significantly widened in many instances (O'Reilly, 1999). Putting the matter crudely, is the transformation of our universities an outcome of 1970s and 1980s consumerist rhetoric, entailing diminished standards, or does it represent an authentic metamorphosis in

British education, with a range of students and subject-matter now deemed **worthy** of inclusion?

There is a snob element in education that sees some areas of study as more 'academic' than others. I once heard of an Oxbridge don who regularly derided degrees in business studies by calling them 'the servile arts'. However, others see a university education as the development of critical awareness, irrespective of the area of study; that it might even be about becoming a 'better' person. In other words, degree level study is about subjecting what one does to critical analysis; it is about learning to think in a certain way. Such 'analytic' definitions cut across the issue of whether this or that subject should be included. Instead, university is seen as a place in which one comes to terms with one's subject, perhaps even with some regard for its social relevance. To that end, many contemporary nurses declare that they no longer work 'in the dark', but are now doing courses to a standard that prepares them to do what they do with greater understanding. So, in such a context, nursing is not only a practical undertaking, but is informed by theoretical and ethical principles. This has resulted in the charge that nursing has become 'too academic', too cut off from basic practice.

Recently, the Council of Deans and Heads of UK University Facilities for Nurses (Martin, 1999a) spoke against separating nursing from higher education and amongst other things, they said this:

'At least 25% of those recruited to pre-registration courses are from people without GCSEs or A levels, so to argue that people who are not academic are excluded is inaccurate'.

This creates as much confusion as it dispels for if a quarter are 'not academic', in the sense that they have no academic qualifications, then what on earth are they doing in a university? More precisely, what, if anything, does this imply about the changed nature of universities? Coupled with the substantial increase in numbers quoted earlier, the absence of even GCSEs among a quarter of nurse entrants suggests a lowering of standards unless, that is, one makes a conceptual leap, whereby so-called 'lowering' of standards is seen as a broadening of the criteria by which we define what higher education is. Some years ago, the novelist (and university lecturer) Kingsley Amis remarked (1991, p. 122) in respect of increasing university numbers, that 'more will mean worse'. It was not, he felt, so much the quality of candidates that was the problem as 'the amount they were required to know in order to get a degree.' For Amis, the 'new age' was about raising the numbers by lowering the standards or, as he caustically put it 'bringing the university into line with the needs of society'.

Theory and practice

The Council of Deans further stated that nursing has been a part of higher education for 'less than two short years', but that, like other disciplines such as the law and medicine, 'it has a long history of criticism about interconnecting practical competence with the critical analysis, which must underpin any quality service'. This statement, I think, contains a detectable sleight of hand. This is because the preoccupation with theory-practice issues in nursing has, in my view, been more conflict ridden—due to the widely different aims and interests of majority and minority nursing groups—a point patently echoed in current debates about nurse education. For, unlike other disciplines, there are some **within** nursing who have doubts about its place within higher education (Williamson, 1998). Naturally, this may reflect concerns about what is being taught—the neglect of practical competencies, for example— but, in any event, there does seem absent in nursing that comfortable, comprehensive assurance, which other disciplines have about their 'proper' place in higher education.

A pertinent criticism by Menzies-Lyth (1988) is that there was little to suggest that nurses from 'the shop floor' of the profession wanted Project 2000, even if, according to Le Var (1997a, 1997b), those at the top did. This hierarchical difference partly accounts for the ongoing uncertainly that still persists, and it was suspicion of such differences that made it possible for the Secretary of State and like-minded others to call for a re-organisation of nurse education in keeping with service oriented requirements.

Why nurses?

Of course, it is not unfair to ask if nurses require a university education. But if this question is going to be asked of nursing, surely there are other groups for whom it could equally be asked. For example, does university level education have a role in the armed services or the police? The probable answer here would be 'yes', but with the proviso that this role would be optional. Options, of course, can lead to divisions and all professions have their divisions. Some lawyers get to be Rumpole of the Bailey: most spend their time conveyancing houses or sorting out messy divorces. Is a degree needed for that? Hardly, for according to my local radio station you can now purchase do-it-yourself packages for divorce, house conveyancing, and making a will. A recent attempt to provide medical diagnoses and treatment via the Internet stalled, although, I suppose, it is early days yet. I am reminded of a character in Alan Bleasdale's play 'The Black Stuff', Yosser Hughes, who, desperate for a job, greeted every employed person he met with the refrain 'Gis' a job. I could do that'.

Plainly, there are walks of life where degrees are unnecessary, even if a growing number of occupations are now 'graduate professions'. Clearly also, forms of cross-validation are needed if occupational roles are to be standardised and, at first sight, it might appear odd if nurses were to opt out of accreditation systems when some of the accredited occupations appear even less plausible for inclusion in academia than nursing. However, matters are made difficult by the tendency in nursing to opt for reforms that have an 'all or nothing' quality about them. Hence, the push to make nursing an **all**-graduate profession with the concomitant 'phasing out' or 'converting' of those whose training was practical. There has always existed a degree of disquiet about the variety of ways by which people qualify as nurses. The sense is of those qualifying by means of a practical route somehow embarrassing the reputation of those with a more exalted entry. Not that multiple or even dual systems would be an easy option. One can imagine the complications that might arise where two newly qualified nurses are assessed for a D Grade post. One has qualified via an academic, university-based programme, whereas the other has come through vocational-based training. Which one will be favoured within a service driven milieu? The academically prepared newcomer is now entering a profession comprised of a system of occupational grades, which take much more account of short-range, practice-based achievements than they do of theory-based academic courses. The tendency of NHS managers to want to fund one and two day courses in selected topics instead of properly accredited, lengthier courses is now well established.

These are some of the conflicts that students quickly pick up and which renders the theory contained in their courses fairly meaningless to them. Unless these fundamental conflicts in respect of the lifetime careers of nurses are resolved, then serious contradictions will persist in respect of the education of nurses and their future role as practitioners. In some respects, these contradictions reflect similar divisions within university education generally, which has become more meritocratic, and a secondary school system that continues to divide along class, economic and, consequently, aspirational lines. But whereas the aspirations of university students generally will be met merely by entering the university system, for nursing students the reality may be more difficult to manage given that the secondary school achievements of many would not normally warrant entry to a university. For that to happen, the universities have had to dumb down their entry criteria and the educational (nursing) elite have had to construct nursing curricula out of all theoretical proportion to what nursing actually is.

Dobson's choice

How odd that so many people, the Secretary of State for Health, Mr. Dobson, included, want to discuss the future of nurse education as if this was the only 'new' occupation to assume academic status. Of course it is not. At the University of Brighton, where I work, there are almost as many students studying business as there are nursing. Now this is interesting because one could equally ask what need there is for business degrees: surely business is about knowing how to make profits? Yet one of the most prestigious degrees in our society is the Master in Business Administration or MBA. Hardly any of these degrees would lack an ethics module as part of their curriculum. Others might protest that the phrase 'business ethics' is an oxymoron **in extremis**. Would, therefore, the Secretary of State for Trade and Industry feel comfortable asking the business community to give up its 'unnecessary' diplomas and degrees in favour of a return to 'learning on the job'? Indeed, the more you think about it the more unusual Mr Dobson's demands become. For example, it is now possible to acquire a degree in retail management, in hotel and tourism, in fashion and photography, equestrian studies, and in agriculture. Oxford University, no less, has for years conferred degrees in agriculture and forestry. Do farmers need a university education in order to farm? It is strange that, while little or no notice was taken of chiropody or fashion as degree level subjects, Mr. Dobson saw fit to publicly denigrate higher education for nurses.

Stereotypes

Our stereotypical notions of what constitutes a university are twofold. On the one hand, there is the image of layabout students, drinking themselves stupid when not soaking up public funds in support of worthless courses. On the other hand, lies Cambridge and Oxford: dreaming spires, languid punting down rivers, and one-to-one tutorials with Nobel Prize winners. The latter, perhaps less so the former, is a far cry from the concrete campuses that heralded an explosion in higher educational provision from the 1960s. However, it is the appropriateness of that overall development, which needs discussing. Seizing upon one group struggling towards some self-recognition of its changing status is both opportunistic and limited. The central issue is the extent to which practice-based occupations require the critical reflection that has traditionally defined academic activity, or whether proportionally more account needs to be taken of the practical requirements of a given occupation.

Gender

In respect of the charge that nurse education should lose its university status, there is, as I have said, the role that gender plays within such assumptions. There is a sadistic element in the knee-jerk reaction of a government that is failing to pick up on the manner by which a right-wing national press (Johnston, 1998; Marrin, 1999; Murray, 1999; Phillips, 1999) has decided (often with discernible virulence) that nurses are no longer 'working' and that their current commitment to higher education merits derision. If nursing were predominantly a male occupation, it is unlikely that these demands to return to the workplace would be made. Nursing has been, especially at the point of delivery, a female preserve and there may be a sense, even within government, that these nurses have 'got above themselves', allowed themselves to be carried away from their traditional preoccupation with nurture, housekeeping, especially hygiene, and, indeed, all things practical.

In the mean time

I suspect that the muddled expectations of (predominantly male) service managers in respect of newly qualified nurses will continue. Likewise, the issue of what should constitute an appropriate curriculum for university level study will continue for some time, albeit, ultimately, the acceptance of dual or multiple portals of entry seems inevitable. However, the divisions implicit in such developments contain the seeds of internal strife within the profession: already we see that higher pay awards are given to special 'consultant nurses'. This, of course, begs the question of what is special within nursing: or is what is meant here, the types of nursing that occur in intensive or high-tech medical settings? The promotion of a small number of university educated nurses to consultant status would offset the disappointment of seeing nurse education revert to a practice-led training. In this way, salaries would again become radically differential, so dodging the, perhaps insurmountable, problem of remunerating an all graduate nursing profession. Could any economy provide the kinds of salaries historically associated with 'the professions' to a broad-based nursing profession? If not, then it is this that will decide, ultimately, many of these issues. In the mean time, nurses must ponder the moral rightness of their claim to professional status against the contention that the practical requirements of their role do not require it.

Psychiatric nursing: a wholly different activity

While these concerns apply to all nurses, an additional set of issues bedevil the psychiatric division. For example, it is a regrettable fact that, on the single occasion when a nursing syllabus gave credence to alternative—social and psychological—concepts of mental disturbance (Mental Health Syllabus, 1982), its implementation lasted all of five years. It says a lot for the commitment of those whose brainchild it was, that this syllabus could be permitted to succumb to something as academically gauche as Project 2000. How could the English National Board (ENB) so rapidly accede to an educational hybrid that, through its 'common foundation' elements, effectively dispossessed psychiatric nursing of its one chance to encourage intellectual dialogue about its philosophy and practice? We will leave it to the social historians to work out why psychiatric nurses lacked the wherewithal to resist the educational blandishments of **Le Projet**.

To assume that they would have wanted an 'opt out', of course, is perhaps doubly naive: the fact is, they didn't. Such acquiescence may be construed as partly due to the historical connection with medical/surgical nursing, as well as divisions within psychiatric nursing itself, particularly on the question of what constitutes mental illness; whether, for instance, social or familial factors are implicated in its causation.

Dissidents

I would like to add my name to the dissidents (see Jackson, 1999) who seek a withdrawal of psychiatric nursing from

Project 2000 and a resumption of direct control over their own three-year syllabus. That this will occur anyway seems certain: the recent shortening of the CFP from 18 months to 12 is not, I imagine, the last we've heard of shortening. To those who would advocate resolving problems from within a Project 2000 perspective, my contention is that the problems are so fundamental (as well as being so obtusely misunderstood by non-psychiatric nurses) that only separation will do the trick. Take but one example: many, many psychiatric patients do not want to be helped and it requires an act of parliament, an act which, outside psychiatric contexts, violates every civil liberty in the book, to enable compulsory treatment to take place. And it is not just a question of patients who are legally certified. As onetime legal advisor to MIND, Larry Gostin (1977) pointed out, who can say what happens in the sitting room of a psychologically distressed person late on a Saturday night in terms of persuading them to come into care, persuading them to accept that the doctors and nurses mean well.

It is this element of compulsion that qualitatively defines psychiatric nursing as a radically different activity to medical/surgical nursing. And it is the kinds of discussion, which such differences require, that becoming involved in Project 2000 prohibited: indeed, inclusion in this 'educational reform' practically swamped the concerns of psychiatric nurses. It did this in two ways: in the first instance, the hyper-emphasis on academia pushed curriculum developers (and their concerns) to the forefront. Second, the Project 2000 initiative consolidated medical-surgical nursing as 'the driving force' behind the reform, especially its common foundation element. Not only did this disenfranchise psychiatric nursing generally, it also made the lot of those who still wished to question its medical assumptions doubly difficult. It specifically disallowed discussion on the nature of psychiatric nursing in the community; whether, for example, community nursing represented more than a mere shift in resources or was, instead, anticipated as a genuine shift in how mentally ill people are supported.

The Project 2000 Syllabus

Educationalists are 'when', 'where', 'how' and 'how often' people, and they become uncomfortable if asked to address questions of 'what'; for example, what is to be taught? If you were waiting for an educational body, like the ENB, to inquire about the content of the psychiatric courses that it validates, you would be waiting a long time. It is hardly surprising, therefore, that many nursing courses emphasise process over substance. In fairness, Project 2000 schemes do invoke holism as an underlying philosophy, as well as espousing a lot of rhetoric about person-centred care. But they have little to say about the nature of mental illness, what our responses to it might be, or the functions that psychiatric practice serve in support of the social and/or political status quo. Not that this has prevented such discussion altogether. Indeed, the conceptual gaps created by Project 2000 prompted different groups (see Keen, 1999) to try to fill it in opposing ways.

One group (Keltner, 1996) seeks to re-establish biology, genetics, and medical technology as core elements of a mental nursing curriculum. These elements, in their turn, are vigorously objected to by others (Barker *et al*, 1998), who seek to retain a more psychological view of the patient's experience. It remains to be seen if, in the long run, either side will 'prevail' or if, as Steve Tilley (1998) believes, elements from both will coalesce into a therapeutic alliance. It is a debate, the nature of which is peculiarly at odds with general nursing, whose commitment needs must be geared towards the pathological/biological status of its patients. Although some protest otherwise, no one takes seriously the view that heart disease is merely the 'absence of health'. Heart disease is not the absence of anything; it is the presence of breathlessness, of not being able to walk, of being in pain. Whatever the holistic ambitions of some nurses in pursuance of health for all, at the heart of general nursing is the treatment of diseases and caring for people who have them.

The elitists among general nurses may protest the seriousness of their newfound humanism. However, theirs is a 'phoney war', a war that asserts holistic health care, but ignores the reality of the rank and file working (frequently under medical pressure) within settings whose primary concerns are people's physical ailments. Naturally, the same is true for nurses working in psychiatric treatment centres: they too incline towards considerations of psychiatric illnesses and their medical treatment. However, for some psychiatric nurses, plausible dissension from medical constructs persists: either they wish to imbue psychotic mental illness with philosophical or social significance, or they seek to extend the remit of psychological 'care' into everyday problems and personal relationships. This 'debate' within psychiatric nursing—wearying as it is to some—nevertheless, possesses a creative tension that is necessary for theoretical development, as well as forming a barrier against the kinds of institutionalisation caused by theoretical disregard. It is, in fact, precisely this debate that characterises what psychiatric nursing is. Yet, because of the educationalist obsession with process, these vital debates are often conducted by small groups of academics within the pages of hardly-read journals, while hardly meriting a mention in student's curricula.:

A unified profession

No greater barrier to progress exists than the belief that what unites the various branches of nursing outweighs their uniquely different properties: this is certainly true for psychiatric nursing. Whether, for example, paediatric nurses would see their role as qualitatively different to that of their adult colleagues is for them to say: assertions to the contrary (Clarke, 1999b) await contradiction. Psychiatric nurses are different; their historical development as an occupation is different; the role of gender in that development is significantly different, as is the differential regard that society has for the various issues, e.g., insanity, which defines their social role. The element of compulsion is but one consequence of society's apprehension about mental illness, particularly since the closure of mental hospitals and the movement of patients into the community. Given that compulsory treatment will shortly receive legal sanction as part of community psychiatric practice, now, more than ever, is there need for an educational space—unconstrained by the reality denials constituting Project 2000 courses—to discuss these issues. To be specific, how does one examine the rightness of defining psychological distress as illness in a context where it is assumed that one belongs in the same grouping as medical-surgical nurses? Of course, the latter group's academic spokespersons insist that such medical involvement is currently a small part of their holistic orientation. However, even the most sober of commentators (Witz, 1994) point to the excessiveness of 'enhanced nursing role' claims, commenting that much nursing development is still predicated on medical and managerial decisions. This is not to say that psychiatric nurses are impervious to medical pressures. But I believe that discussion about alternative (non-medical) concepts of mental illness are more plausible, more realistic in psychiatry than for general medicine. This scope is dramatically less than it was, say, thirty years ago, and medical aficionados within psychiatric nursing anticipate further lessening still. However, comfort may be taken from the fact that voluntary users of psychiatric services are rarely enamoured of their medical nature (Coleman and Smith, 1997), and unsurprisingly so since many are compelled to accept treatment. Of course, satisfied customers are less likely to speak out and no doubt there are many who have benefited from physical treatments. Nevertheless, issues like these require a wider arena than that provided by medicine alone: these issues are more obviously social and political in character. The continued diversion of psychiatric nursing educators into the exhausting business of delineating Project 2000 schemes is a distraction from more relevant debates about mental 'illness' and the political, social, and philosophical functions that its diagnosis and treatment deserves in our society.

The future

There has been a perceptible shift in favour of recapturing old educational ground: the CFP has been shortened to one year and, in many cases, what remains is 'common foundation' in name only. For instance, the recommendation that students from the different branches be provided with CFP teaching, pertaining to their speciality is being implemented. In addition, the link with practice has been reinvigorated and nurse education is now in reversal, from having been theory, to again being practice-led. For most nurses, this is how matters are likely to remain. That being so, serious questions will need to be asked about the appropriateness of basic nurse education staying within the university system. Without doubt, a minority will adamantly cling to their position within higher education, and these may well become the spokespersons for the profession, whether within educational or practising contexts. Such differentials in professional standing will—as is already happening—lead to differences in pay, and it may well be that the Halsbury concept of curtailing pay differences will need to be discarded. In general, nursing should be looking at how to accommodate diversity within its ranks: the notion of a unified profession is probably now dead.

3
The geography of care

Prologue

*T*he late Maxwell Jones, a pioneer of the therapeutic community movement, always said that it was important to note **where** psychiatry was practised. For example, he did not think that a humane psychiatry was possible within the grounds of general hospitals. But, of course, it was precisely to these hospitals that acute psychiatry moved following the virtual closure of the mental hospitals, and it is the physical, social, and therapeutic situations of these patients that constitutes my area of concern.

The geography of psychiatric care is important for several reasons; for example, studies leading to changes in psychiatric practice have invariably taken social construction as their starting point. Analyses of mental hospitals, for instance, began by examining 'the hospital as a social system' (Belknap, 1956; Rapoport, 1960; Shoenberg, 1980) and, in the main, they ended up condemning what they saw as endemic institutionalisation. However, institutionalisation apart, what was startling at the time was the sheer fact of hospitals being subject to social analysis and the remarkable conflicts that these studies revealed. While these exposed conflicts took various forms, basic to most of them was the tendency for both staff and patient behaviours to become deeply entrenched and resistant to change.

Institutionalisation gripped the mental hospitals, although the rigidity of its grasp varied, again as a function of geography. By the 1950s, the Victorian-built hospitals could be divided mainly into three categories, although not entirely, in respect of their location. A small number had, through the leadership of enlightened medical superintendents, become fairly liberal, open hospitals. The first of these, Dingleton Hospital, was located in Melrose, a tranquil rural setting in Scotland. A second, much larger group of hospitals, set within rural communities, had also achieved a fair measure of democracy for their patients. A third group, almost all of which were situated in or near large cities, were the most restrictive: these were the so-called 'bins', the last, dreariest, obstinate remnants of Dickensian England.

The current crop

For anyone who dislikes institutions, it would be nice to think that they are safely gone, although to believe that would be foolish. The fact is, the essentials of asylum/hospital life remain, albeit in various new and sometimes beguiling forms. For instance, their custodialism is presently subsumed within forensic and challenging behaviour units and, ironically, many of these continue to inhabit the grounds of the old mental hospitals. These custodial units are the hinterland of psychiatric nurses, the end-point of their historic utility as the policing arm of psychiatry, where the alleged (sometimes real) aggressive propensities of 'the mad' are kept at a safe distance from the populace.

Andrew Scull (1996) quite rightly points out that the closure of mental hospitals, and the subsequent move of patients into the community, occurred in the absence of any careful evaluation of the relative merits of either: within this vale of unknowing, a supercilious depiction of the hospitals as a kind of socio-terrorism was matched by the supposed attractions of the community as a more liberating form of care. In fact, little community infrastructure existed to cater for the mentally ill and no evidence existed to show that such people were welcome in the first place. What surprises is that anyone could have imagined an easy transition of patients from a system whose purpose (in part) was to contain the apprehensions of a general public, unaccustomed to the idea of the mentally ill living next door. Now it was proposed to bring these patients, if not next door, then certainly into the hub of local communities.

The 'totality' of mental hospitals, to use Goffman's (1961) phrase, had lessened by the 1950s. For example, the 'open door movement' was underway, although behind this movement, a hidden trickery ensured that patients who were absconders, or seen as anti-social, continued to be confined.

Many of the conventional mores of hospital life were simply carried over into the community when these hospitals began to discharge their patients in large numbers. By and large, most localised psychiatric units did not acquire new or different ways of doing things, but continued much the same as before. It would be absurd to suggest that they took no account of their changed circumstances and, on the whole, the social lives of some patients have improved.

In the main, however, the medicalisation of psychological distress proceeded apace, as it continues to do. Having said that, the main impediment to a fuller transfer of medical control into the community was the need to manage anti-social or even dangerous patients. Unsurprisingly, as political concerns grew about the conduct of some of these patients, so the policing function of psychiatry needed to be extended. Important aspects of that extension are the Community Treatment Orders (DoH, 1999b), which permit forced treatments in 'the community'. Predictably, the psychiatric professions, partly because they are divided on these issues, were unable to forestall what some saw as a violation of patient's civil rights.

Zone of autonomy

The idea of patients living beneficially in the community only makes sense if their discharge from hospital leads to an increase in their autonomy. Mentally ill people have never been regarded as possessing autonomy in its usual sense. Mental health legislation that allows for compulsory treatments derives from assumptions that mental patients have lost the capacity for rational thought. Therefore, under existing legislation, if a discharged patient used his newfound 'autonomy' to refuse medication, he could then be re-admitted and compulsorily treated. The legislation currently proposed is that treatment is carried out without hospital admission, presumably in the patient's home. Thomas Szasz once said (BBC, 1989) that patients are hospitalised and treated, not because they have problems, but because other people have problems with **them**. Szasz's claim is far from the whole truth, but I do think that it represents part of a truth. The annoyance caused to family or friends by abnormal behaviours helps explain why the social separation of mentally ill people is often seen as a worthwhile move. It is also something that is dependent on social class, education, and the ability to pay, as well as where the annoyance occurs. Diagnosis is a kind of social arbitration, whereby certain behaviours are no longer to be seen as socially credible: the complaint of relatives or social workers that someone's behaviour is socially intolerable is validated. Naturally, there is more to it than this or every teen-ager in the land could be diagnosed insane by frantic parents and power mad doctors. Why this does not happen is due to the nature of the peculiarities of affected individuals that seems to call for some sort of extraordinary reaction, such as medical intervention. Here is how Anthony Clare (BBC, 1989) puts it:

> 'There are disturbances which so effect mental functioning that civilised societies say the responsibility of this man or woman for what has happened is impaired, and is impaired in such a way as, therefore, to suggest to one society or another that they may be dealt with differently'.

But, at least, hospitalisation signified that those being coer-cively treated were being removed from the everyday settings within which the general rules of ethical and social engage-ment applied. This seemed to acknowledge that a transforma-tion in the affected individual's status was needed, if a forced treatment was to follow. Goffman (1961) argued that complex and prolonged social procedures attended hospital admis-sion, so as to legitimise this transformation. Goffman, always critical of institutions, described admission procedures as 'degradation ceremonies' whose effect was to strip people of fundamental elements of their personhood: their resultant patient status rendering them less entitled to the normal pro-tection and dignities of the law and society. Admission proce-dures were almost always the responsibility of nurses. How cognisant they would have been of Goffman's strictures is debatable. Almost all would, I think, have been puzzled by his interpretation, although, if pressed, would have had difficulty denying the dehumanising effects of a range of hospital procedures, not just admission. However, they would have defended their actions on the grounds that these patients were mentally ill and in need of treatment. 'Degradation ceremonies' were less to do with demeaning individuals and more about the creation and maintenance of treatment milieus in which normative rules of human engagement no longer applied (see *Chapter 6*).

Crystallising consent

Today, psychiatric beds are a rare commodity and admitting people to hospital is not always an option. The imposition of Community Treatment Orders (CTOs) crystallises issues of consent and psychiatric management, because they address the nagging problem of finding a mechanism by which psychiatry imposes its policing role. These orders seek to solve the question of how to forcibly treat people, but without the proviso of hospital admission. Does this matter? Might not CTOs be a more economical way of managing awkward social behaviour, more humane inasmuch as patients will continue living at home, while being medicated? Possibly. What CTOs also confirm, however, is that living in the community is not an indication of free and equitable citizenship status, since excluded from that status is the right to refuse treatment. In effect, the community becomes a virtual hospital with all of the old powers and responsibilities of asylum life intact.

From hospital to community

Macleod Clark *et al* (1996) refer to figures from Bosanquet and Gerard (1985) to the effect that about 50% of charge and staff nurses work in non-hospital settings. This is an interesting statistic in itself, but it seems to be doing much more than is apparent at first sight: in effect, it seems to be staking a claim for the validity of community based practice. Since, at the moment, elements within general nursing seek to transform themselves into a community-based preventative practice, a few words about the problematic experiences of psychiatric nurses, who have already made the move into 'the community', might prove timely, even enlightening.

Hart (1994) puts the number of psychiatric nurses who work in hospitals at 85% of the total and this seems more accurate and not just intuitively so. Specifically, about 7500 operate as Community Psychiatric Nurses (CPNs) with perhaps 66 000 continuing to work within treatment centres (Brooker and White, 1998). Admittedly, many of these treatment centres are now situated in the high-street: defining them as 'care in the community', however, only works if you accept that community care is defined, either in whole or in part, by geography. I imagine that geography does play a modest part since, with the closure of the mental hospitals, considerable movement of patients into the community has occurred. Such movement has not as yet significantly affected the nature of the therapy or care delivered, and the tendency is for psychiatric units to continue to work along medicalised lines.

With the closure of the large hospitals, the relocation of wards closer to the hub of ordinary communities might have been expected to encourage more 'normalised' systems of living within them: perhaps just 'being there' might eventually bring about such changes. It is early days, after all. For the moment, the point seems to be missed (by many) that there is a significant difference between nurses who happen to work in the community, as opposed to those seeking to implement community care (White, 1998). The latter approach hints at disenchantment with concepts of illness and perhaps a greater consideration of how social events may influence illness development, or alleviate its chronicity. Allowing that the numbers of psychiatric nurses swamp those of medical psychiatrists, and allowing that nursing had taken on a strong person-centred dimension, it might seem feasible to expect that they would have attempted even a modest revision of their traditional medical role. Yet, while this did occur in patches (Cole 1990), by and large, it has been the medical approach that has prevailed.

The truth about schizophrenia

The medical explanation for schizophrenia is predictably straightforward: it is an illness. Of course, the medics can go a bit deeper than this on schizophrenia: they can outline its bio-chemical basis and this outline is persuasive in its own right. Indeed, it is the tangential character of the medical outline, its linear elegance, the completeness of its form that carries great force. As one nurse-lecturer comments, the medical model is attractive because it is 'nice and logical and its scientific and you can do it in school beautifully' (Davies, 1998: p103). We can outline one of its versions schematically:

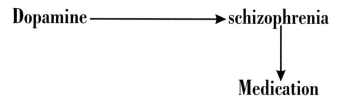

Figure 3.1: The dopamine hypothesis and schizophrenia

The 'explanation' runs like this: an excess of dopamine results in psychosis and, indeed, people with schizophrenia do appear to have too much dopamine. This is supported from post-mortem data where the number of dopamine receptors is markedly increased. In addition, the effectiveness of anti-psychotic drugs is related to their antagonistic effect on dopamine. As Fortinash and Holoday-Worret (2000) point out, while the evidence as a whole is inconclusive, the 'Dopamine Hypothesis' continues to generate interest and research. It has also, more pertinently, taken on something of the status of a truism within conventional psychiatric practice. I shall now contrast this model with another, this time drawn from social theory (see *Figure 3.2*).

In this model, each circle represents either a family member or someone involved with a family during the process of diagnosis or treatment of one of its members. For example, CP stands for consultant psychiatrist, F for father and P for

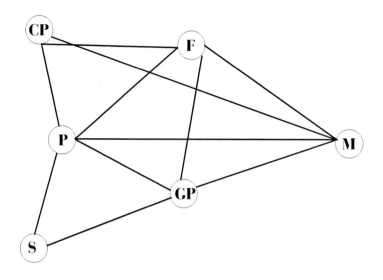

Figure 3.2: A social model of the genesis of schizophrenia

patient. You can see that the circles (people) are linked by lines each of which represents a unit of communication between them. This diagram represents the minimum of exchanges and the reader is asked to consider what a day's conversation would look like for such a group. One can imagine the difficulties of entering such a maelstrom—as a CPN, for example—where, in effect, one becomes (just) another line in the matrix. One way of countering the unwanted effects of such intrusions might be to use a family therapy approach, where an outside 'commentator' monitors the family/therapeutic sessions via a one-way mirror system and communicates any therapeutic biases (via an ear-piece) to the therapist directly involved. Cumbersome, perhaps, but a more democratic, less didactic, way of structuring mental health interventions in respect of some problems. However, the point is not to affirm the validity of either a medical or social approach, so much as to suggest that the **persuasiveness** of the medical view is linked to its linear, accessible and thus more assimilative form. Contrariwise, therapies derived from social theories of mental illness are less likely to attract nurses, since they lack the conceptual clarity of the medical explanation and it is this explanation that sustains most settings dealing with psychologically distressed people.

Defining approaches

There was a time when these two approaches would have been defined in terms of where they took place: the family model as part of a community approach, perhaps, with the linear model located within hospital or other treatment settings. However, this is not, and never has been, the case. Incongruously, most social experiments in psychiatry (Cooper, 1961; Jones, 1982) originated within institutions. Indeed, community psychiatric practice evolved from hospital practice, albeit, as noted, there are, regrettably, too many instances where this shows. The therapeutic community movement took root inside a British mental hospital at a time when these hospitals were already earmarked for closure. The Gadarene rush of patients from the rapidly closing hospitals led to an avoidance of the problems of patients who continued to live within those that remained.

A rhetoric of 'community care' had beguiled many into a belief that mental hospitals were, by definition, bad for people; a dubious notion, but made sensible by the institutionalisation that had corrupted them. Undoubtedly, their overcrowding, as well as the 'inborn and irredeemable' beliefs about mental illness held by the staff, was inimical to decent care. Yet, to assume that their closure would bring about a changed conceptualisation of mental illness and its treatment was unrealistic. Patients continued to be medicalised, although now living in 'the community' and, under current law, Gray (1998a) has detailed how patients living in the community can be thoroughly degraded in the process of forcibly treating them.

Legal mischief

Like most people, I imagined that government policies were carefully thought through, that the administration of law was fair and that governments would inform us about diseased food as naturally as they would ask for our votes. No more. Now I know that public officials do not always act on 'the facts', but might sometimes tell us what they want us to hear. Even so, it was a surprise to discover that the number of killings by mentally disordered people is half what it was 20 years ago (Nursing Times, 1999a) and that, indeed, these 'low rates' had been known for some time. Howitt (1998), for instance, reports a number of studies largely confirming this, while implicating the media in contriving the kinds of negative imagery often associated with mentally ill people living in the community.

In the case of mental health, 'the community' has become, for many, a byword for every fantasy imaginable: a place of murder and unease, of loss of control, humiliation, vagrancy, and dispossession. The tabloids have highlighted every transgression, 'defining' each attack as **characteristic** of mental illness, specifically schizophrenia.

For those directly affected, the consequences of violence are tragic beyond words. Yet, as the relatives of victims' point out, the answer is not about blaming individual patients, rather is it about examining how the social order might be better organised to take account of changes in the provision of patient services. The National Schizophrenia Fellowship (1999), for example, points to shortages of accommodation, lack of employment, and poor crisis management as all needing urgent attention. Yet few would deny that funding services in the community—commensurate with the loss of services represented by the hospital closures—has been generally poor. In place of funding or, more accurately, in addition to modest funding, various legislative changes are proposed that seek to 'tighten up' a community care, which is perceived as out of the control of the professions. That being so, proposals that some patients be compelled to accept treatments against their will may be avoiding more complex (and expensive) alternatives as a matter of political expediency.

While the standard of community care has been discussed many times, the question of who is or is not fit to live freely in society has not. Traditionally, we relied on the asylum/hospital as both a custodial and therapeutic response to recalcitrant patients, and this plausibly dealt with the question of civil rights insofar as detained patients, treated against their will, were at least judged to be unable to live safely in society. Legislation provided for their detention and treatment provided they were a danger to themselves or to others. It is asking a lot of professionals that they impose treatment regimes in a context where the patient continues to be regarded as fit to live in society. It is especially worrying if CPNs are going to be required to impose force. According to Mr Paul Boateng, current proposals do not 'entail, in practice, distressed patients being held down against their will and forcibly injected over their own kitchen tables'. However, while there is much in the government's White Paper, 'Modernising Mental Health Services' (DoH, 1998) that is good, it also contains much that is confusing and, ultimately, oppressive. Witness, for example, its contention that 'a modern legal framework must offer the flexibility to tackle unacceptable risk to personal or public safety wherever it occurs' as well as Mr Boeteng's statement that 'the law must make it clear that non-compliance with treatment programmes is not an option'.

And after the violent act, what?

Undoubtedly, in many cases, compulsion will not extend beyond persuasion. However, bearing in mind that treatment in these cases means physical treatment, and allowing that some patients will refuse absolutely, it seems inevitable that physical force will, on occasions, be required. The logic of the proposed changes leaves little option. That being the case, the prospect of entering someone's home and forcibly 'treating' them, the police cuffing them prior to their being injected—oral force-feeding of pills is surely not an option—

and, in a context, where the person continues to live freely in society (and all that that implies) is just bizarre. And after the violent act, what? How will the CPN respond when the patient says 'shame'. We are talking about free people here, people who happen not to want treatment: whose intransigence, such as it is, is not necessarily a symptom of illness.

To be free is to be able to choose: CTOs in effect say: 'you are semi-free: free to live in your community, but not quite, not without medication'. In effect, the provisions of the asylum/hospital are extended to society at large: CTOs establish a virtual asylum whose boundaries are fixed as effectively by statute as by bricks and mortar. One doubts if even an Erving Goffman, with his vivid capacity to invoke the nightmarish properties of 'total institutions', could have anticipated a therapeutic bureaucracy of such widespread proportions.

In support

Compulsion, of course, has its supporters. From a sociological standpoint, Peter Morrall (1998) argues that psychiatric nursing is a quasi profession, which consistently avoids owning up to its historical task of 'policing the mad'. There is much in what he says, although he appears to ignore undercurrents of resistance to custodialism (for example the therapeutic community movement), as well as the 'carer' versus 'controller' dialectic endemic to forensic psychiatric provision (Clarke, 1996). Morral's problematic analysis—sufficiently problematic for the psychiatric nursing fraternity to have all but ignored it—goes to the core of what nurses are for in a modern society. Historically, their combined role of gaoler and 'carer' is unquestionable, although it could be argued that much has happened in the last 20 (post hospital) years to have changed this.

In 1999, the National Schizophrenia Fellowship (NSF) declared that the debate on compulsory treatments is misplaced, rather, we should be pressuring governments into providing better all round care. Indeed, a survey of NSF users, carers and professionals resulted in a majority **favouring** compulsion. Interestingly, its ethnic minority members were more wary of the implications. While the views of the NSF are important, they too easily ignore the downsides of institutional provision (Martin, 1984; Stanley *et al*, 1999), the tendency for good intentions to fall prey to corporate need, and professional pressures.

The neglected pragmatics of enforcement

A serious lack of pragmatics attends discussions about enforced treatments. Most, for example, assume a fairly compliant patient, but, outside hospital contexts, patients may be quite resistive. The hospital was there to be got out of: co-operation brought its rewards. The community, however, is open-ended and so compulsion orders may have nowhere to go, but into the invisible peace and quiet of habitual enforcement. The asylum/hospital was a concrete expression of society's response to difficult people, a focal point for ongoing debates on the adequacies or otherwise of psychiatric practice. Within the more disseminated anonymity of community provision, the repressive instinct is more, not less, likely to flourish. Responding to professional boasts that most hospitalised patients in Britain were 'voluntary', Larry Gostin (1977) suggested that we may never know what lies behind the voluntary status of patients who, in their own front rooms, have 'agreed' that hospital admission would be best for **all** concerned.

Will the 'new' information on diminished violence by mentally ill people give cause for hesitation? I somehow doubt it. Fear and finance are the spurs that drive this legislative reform. A government desirous of being seen to 'do something' is unlikely to begin educating the public with the uncomfortable fact that dangers are less than they imagined.

Duty to care

If concepts of dangerousness are inapplicable, then, irrespective of the White Paper's (DoH, 1998) references to 'risk to self or others', some will assume (as they do now) a concept of 'duty to care'. This difficult-to-legislate-for concept can justify treating anybody, from the dying to the unhygienic. Its beauty, however, is that it may just as properly be utilised in supporting patients' refusals of treatment. Having said that, for those who believe that illness determines all, we may confidently expect that 'duty to care' will, given time, disavow patient's choices as invalid because 'lacking insight'.

The ambiguity of mental illness is what excuses biological psychiatry from considering the demands of affected individuals' as valid. This kind of psychiatry takes as read that physical pathology is pretty much all that matters. Concepts of biological defect are the engine room that drive CTOs.

A way of practising psychological nursing (and medicine) has never been so urgently required as now. Few may argue with the supervision of patients who are a danger to self or others. The operative word, however, is 'might'. Is it right, for instance, that someone with a mental illness who has stopped taking their medication should be coerced into taking it again because the professionals **anticipate** deterioration? How might patients be 'helped' within a therapeutic alliance that refuses to respect their decisions or acknowledge their capacity to weigh up (rightly or wrongly) the pros and cons of their taking decisions about themselves and others?

It is said that the imposition of treatments will occur only rarely, as a last resort. However, as Tony Heath (1998) says, that it will occur at all will go some way towards defining what a mental health nurse is. Equally, if it is going to be such a rare event, why the need to enshrine it in law? Either I'm missing something along the line, or we're not being told the full story.

In the following example, a young black man, calling himself John Baptist, is subjected to a psychiatric regime as malevolent as anything described by Goffman (1961) Foucault (1971) or Fanon (1967). Filmed by the BBC (Minders, 1995) the 'responsible medical officer' for John Baptist, challenged about his diagnosis, replies:

'Schizophrenia is a complex disorder which is characterised by strange beliefs which we call delusions, strange experiences called hallucinations—hearing voices talking about you. He's

never talked about hearing voices. And he's never given evidence of what's called thought disorder, but I have no doubt that this is a schizophrenic illness'.

The nurse

As for the nurse —intensive outreach worker—most closely involved in this case, her main contribution to the diagnostic/treatment process, as Gray (1998) shows, is to support notions of 'hygiene', 'order' and 'responsibility' as evidence of 'well-being and good health'. On her way to a first meeting with John, the outreach worker states:

'My primary thing is to get a relationship going with him but I'm not prepared to compromise the fact that I think he's got a mental illness'.

Within minutes of meeting John she is heard on the sound-track saying:

'Money's important to him. At the minute side-effects are extremely important to him. His privacy and his self-respect are important to him and I don't think me believing he has a mental illness has to compromise those things.

Exactly who is asking for these compromises is not made clear. Her reiteration of the phrase 'mental illness' is also notable. Some minutes later, she persuades John to apply for a bus pass.

Nurse: 'You can get a bus pass if you are mentally or physically disabled in some way. Now most of the clients I work with, because we feel that they have a mental illness, they are entitled to a bus pass, but you would have to sign something to say that that you, you are suffering from a mental illness and I know the other week when we talked about it, you weren't happy to do that. So, I mean, I believe you're suffering from a mental illness'.

John: 'You can get me a bus pass'?

Nurse: 'Would that be all right?'

John: 'Yes, you can get me a bus pass'.

Nurse: 'OK. That's the bit where it says 'My disability is'. Now, my feeling, and I know you disagree with it, is that you do have a mental illness that causes you some problems and certainly, at the moment, the treatment for what we feel to be your mental illness is causing you great problems because its causing you a lot of shakes and difficulties'.

John: 'Yea, Yea'.

Nurse: 'It says there 'I am permanently and substantially disabled' which is a very heavy thing to say. Now, I think, at the minute, you are suffering from a mental illness and that therefore you are disabled, not least your having problems with the treatment your getting for it'.

John: 'It's OK. It's OK.'

Nurse: 'Its difficult isn't it?'

John: 'Yes.'

John reluctantly signs the document.

Gray (1998a) comments that in this exchange the patient 'is made to feel the interior of his disease and the stigma that this holds for orthodox morality': in Goffman's (1961) terms, a 'degradation ceremony' has occurred in which the patient's self has been thoroughly mortified.

Hygiene

Suman Fernando (1991) points to the manner by which 'order and hygiene' can be negatively invoked against members of ethnic minority groups who are seen as mentally ill as, historically, it was part and parcel of derogatory attitudes towards working class people. Asked by a tribunal member why John Baptist should be hospitalised if, as his consultant has stated, 'he is not a nuisance to his neighbours and clearly looks after himself', the senior registrar replies:

'Yes...Umm...,I can't dispute that. But I think there's more to well-being and good health than simple physical safety, in terms of...hmmm...feeding, clothing, washing.'

In other words, here is someone, still living in the community, being treated as an object, deciphered (and ultimately incarcerated) because a doctor is distraught at his perceived lack of hygiene, which she then reconstructs as a mental illness. The point is, it is not the geography of care that matters and claims by pro-medical nurses (Gournay and Brooking, 1994) that post nineteen-sixties CPN practice had somehow 'lost its medical way', somehow exchanged its biological birthright for a counselling repartee, gave rise to serious misconceptions about community care. What actually occurred is that, with the closure of the asylums, previously hospitalised schizophrenic patients were now decanted into the community and the asocial reactions of a small number of them became politically intolerable. The fact of many CPNs not having had schizophrenic patients on their caseloads was no longer acceptable in political terms, since they would now be needed to 'plug a gap' created by the closures. Research that sought to draw attention to CPN practice as a non-psychotic 'counselling' activity seemed unaware of the political implications of its findings. By advocating a re-jigging of the work of existing CPNs in the direction of psychotic patients, this research indirectly affirmed the politico-managerial correctness of 'making do with what you have got'. The notion of campaigning for more CPNs was never a serious runner. Once again, an alliance with medical ideology prevented a more comprehensive (nursing) assessment of people's needs in society and of how nurses might respond to those needs.

Evidence base

It's an uncomfortable truth that medical explanations precipitate institutionalisation probably because they obviate any need to inquire further. They assume—admittedly in the wrong (usually over-enthusiastic) hands—a 'science has now shown' veneer. The insecure desire of some psychiatric nurses to latch on to medical information—be it molecular genetics or biochemistry—ignores that such information is fragmented and contradictory, often unstable over time, as well as being influenced by culture in important ways. The cult of 'evidence-based care' derives from a view of life that takes as read that all human knowledge is conducive to forms of factual communication. Implicit in current discussions about the role of evidence is that professional work, which cannot (or will not) generate quantitative data, is just not good enough. It's as if, having cornered small areas of patient care that lend themselves to quantitative discussion, they then castigate nurses who fail to match this evidence-based standard. Absence of evidence, however, is not evidence of absence (of distress) and attempts to restrict psychiatric nursing to defined categories of (so-called serious and enduring) patients are misguided. Further, the brutal devotion to medicalised responses of some psychiatric nurses, as well as their strangely contradictory beliefs about how hygiene constitutes 'the good life', is disturbing.

Neighbourhood cleansing

Neighbourhood cleansing is in the air. The homeless, poor, alcoholic, and 'down and out' are an eye-sore: proposed legislation to allow compulsory treatment of psychiatric patients in the community is but a legal sanction of a spreading intolerance of 'street people'. I have been accused of hysteria (Atkinson, 1999) in drawing attention to the new brutalism (Clarke, 1999c) inherent within psychiatric nursing's rediscovery of the supposed blessings of neurobiology, psychoactive drugs, brain scan technology, and the curious reluctance to challenge what, in my view, is oppressive legislation.

I have made the point that CPNs have not demonstrated their clinical independence from hospital derived medical practice. Professor Kevin Gournay (1996: p194), for example, states that 'pharmacological approaches to serious mental illness are widening all the time and CPNs will become more important in this area as prescribers of medication'. How exactly one reconciles such a medical extension of responsibilities within an enhanced nursing role is beyond me. I had thought that the nursing response would more appropriately mediate between medical prescriptions and patient's responses to them: it is hardly the nurse's responsibility to 'sell' prescriptive drugs to patients. In the case of John Baptist— which I hold to be a not untypical representation—the failure of a community outreach team to move beyond a startlingly narrow pathology and hospital derived framework was stunning. Equally, their smug assumption that, although John was not a danger to anyone, including himself, he, nevertheless, required forced hospitalisation was perplexing. Summing up John's community treatment, Dr Suman Fernando, asked by a Mental Health Tribunal to give a 'second opinion', said:

> 'I don't doubt that the intensity of these feelings would be reduced and, in medical terms he would be seen to improve: strictly medical terms, I mean narrow medical terms, if you see, and he'll then have to take his medication each time. If he stops he'll relapse and he'll be given medication again and gradually he will become a chronic patient. He'll be sort of zombie like from time to time. He'll lose his enthusiasm about life. In the past he would have been institutionalised in hospital, now he'll be institutionalised in the community, perhaps going to a day-centre, stitching things together or something like that and he'll be a...success.'

4
Closely observed students?

Du r ing my career I have often been required to invigilate examinations. Although, invariably, a tedious undertaking, there was the odd occasion when I thought that I had observed something suspicious going on between candidates: an arm-span between adjacent candidates that was just a little too wide for comfort perhaps, or maybe some shifty looks which indicated that something was amiss. I usually attributed such things to a misinterpretation. In any event, I would have needed to be really sure: there would be little point in thinking I had seen something and it would never do to act on suspicion; one would have to be indisputably sure. These were my views, long before the events I describe here took place. I like to think that I had always believed that I would never act against a candidate without grave reason. But I did, and the reason I did is because on a particular day, during a particular examination, I was categorically sure that I witnessed one candidate pass information to another.

The humanistic impulse

Before describing what took place, I should point out that this is not just a story of alleged transgression, but is also about how the truth of a case can be mocked when false dogma and its rhetoric take the place of honest inquiry; when a set of artificial principles, derived from a counselling orthodoxy, are substituted for the everyday ethics and rules of engagement by which we live our lives. It is also about the demise of tradition, as well as a loss of respect for authority.

From the 1950s and onwards, the American writer Carl Rogers (1951) had preached a form of 'being with' other people—both in real life and in professional relationships—which, at its core, contained an absolute belief in the goodness of mankind. So-called Rogerian, or humanistic, counselling became the cornerstone of human encounter groups and relationship therapy mushroomed. Rogers' teaching consisted of a series of precepts (which he called Core Conditions) of which non-judgementalism was one. According to his theory—in my view an ethical prescription, not a theory—one exhibited towards one's clients an unconditional positive regard at all times. In addition, one also possessed empathy in the sense of experiencing or seeing matters from the perspective of whoever was being counselled, or 'being with' at a given time.

It would be difficult to underestimate the influence of this so-called 'person-centred' counselling: certainly, within nursing, it won hands down against all competing 'philosophies'; a plethora of textbooks, as well as nursing courses, insisted that students exhibit positive regard for their patients, be prepared to form relationships with them, give them time, space, and so on.

The downside of this is difficult to pinpoint because superficially beguiling. Rogers argued that people are inherently good so that, if given a choice, they will always choose 'personal growth' and 'fulfilment'. Implicit in his, and his followers, teaching is that evil is something that can be 'worked on': people are not bad, but have simply not experienced the kinds of conditions that might make them good. In practical terms, the most common outcome of this philosophy is that it leads to a playing down of personal responsibility. A philosophy that takes as a first principle a position of never judging anyone else, and obliges a person to empathise emphatically with another viewpoint is, at the least, questionable.

Impressionable students could be forgiven for lacking a critical viewpoint on this. That representatives of the English National Board (ENB) should similarly lack a critical acuity in respect of such a 'philosophy' is a measure of the Board's continuing preoccupation with process rather than content. The ENB could be seen to have championed this 'relationship-forming' approach to the point where examination candidates, who failed to state that they would form relationships with their clients, who failed to state, for example, that they would employ a 'therapeutic use of self', would run the risk of failing. Of course, none of this is unconnected with the obsession that western society has visited upon 'the individual' and his or her rights in recent times. It seems hard to deny that this concern with individualism has accompanied a general deterioration in social standards, a situation reflected in the high standing currently allotted to relativism.

What actually took place

While invigilating an ENB Examination for Registered Nurses, I saw a candidate pass his question paper to another candidate sitting beside him. She read from this paper while he looked around absentmindedly. I observed this for some seconds and became so convinced that something was amiss that I acted. At the finish of the examination, together with my Senior Tutor, I confronted the two students with my observations. I told them that I had seen the passage of the paper from one to the other, had seen the other read from it, and that I was reporting this to the ENB as a 'serious infringement' in the examination room.

I thought that everything, from then on, would be 'routine'. After all, what are invigilators for? A report of misconduct is made to a governing body who then asks some expeditious questions and that is that. Accordingly, I submitted my Report, confidently awaited their questions, but was instead informed that a delegation would visit me 'to make further enquiries'. Whereas I had assumed an 'open and shut case', clearly I was wrong. In the event, the Board's visitors were polite but persistent. Understandably, they asked to see the examination room and, although, as they left, they seemed happy enough, I could sense they were vaguely dissatisfied.

Later, I was told there would be further enquiries and that, possibly, the students involved might have 'a point of view'. At this I became angry and shouted (at an ENB member) that this was absurd. 'I am the presiding invigilator', I said, 'and this is ridiculous. My word on these matters is the Board's word. Are you proposing to investigate yourselves?' In measured tones, they advised that both students would question me in the presence of a Commission of Inquiry in a 'genuine attempt to get at the truth'. Suffice it to say that the quality of my response to this suggestion led to its' speedy withdrawal. However, they insisted, portions of my statement would be given to the students and a Commission of Inquiry would be convened. Embarrassed and confused, I was of course obligated to attend.

First time

This was the first (reported) incident of 'cheating' in British nursing history and it focussed attention, revealingly, on the practice of invigilation whose conventions, I had assumed, were well defined. Timeless student jokes about hiding notes in lavatory cisterns or smuggling materials into examination rooms always seemed to be fuelled by the imagined thrill of being caught. Of course, the evocative power of invigilation stemmed, in part, from endless cycles of uneventful examinations: in other words, 'getting caught' was, for both student and invigilator, an unlikely fantasy. The validity of invigilation depended on the decreasing—but still prevalent—need to maintain the classical 'three-hour written paper'. To the extent that such examinations needed to be executed in the timeworn manner (i.e. without candidate's notes or other assistance), then the invigilation role seemed a given. Today's continuously assessed students are perhaps less conscious of examinations, as the summative events determining their progress or failure. More relevant to them, perhaps, is the much greater emphasis on so-called experiential learning and assessment. Non-examination assessment is predicated on learner-centredness as a viable educational method, which no doubt it is in many cases. However, it, too, has helped shift balances of power and, perhaps, even authority in respect of teaching and learning. If students are presented with schedules of learning whereby such things as individual reflection and peer review are given undue weight—and I feel that nurse education has veered too far from notions of collective responsibility—then it can hardly surprise if the re-imposition of traditional values—albeit in this instance with a jolt—produces a measure of anger and confusion.

In a relativist context, it is not surprising that two nursing students were stunned when confronted (judgmentally) with the consequences of their actions in one of the few areas of education where absolute authority prevails, the examination room. On the other hand, what was unexpected was how this relativism was carried over into the inquiry itself, with a determined effort to value every perception as equally valid. The retention of a 'counter-culture' mentality (with attendant '1960s' language) among nurse teachers, has not gone unnoticed (Burnard, 1990). However, it beggars belief that such thinking could govern an investigation into the factual statements of a presiding invigilator about events occurring in an examination.

On the 14th April 1993, the Commission began its questioning of me as presiding invigilator. Needless to say, all names have been changed.

The Commission

The Chairman: This is Helen Storey and Frank Mitchell and I believe we have met, Kevin Brown just to remind you.

We would just wish to ask from you to give us, as full an account of the actual things that occurred on that day as you can. We have read a copy of your report and I suppose it is just now to check out some of those issues with you.

Just a little bit about where we stand in terms of any decisions made or whatever. What we are seeing is that it is the College's responsibility to prove beyond any doubt that collusion and cheating actually occurred and, if there are issues that are vague or can be interpreted in alternative ways, we think our position at the moment is that we will veer towards those people who have been accused of the cheating. So, we principally see it as your position to prove to us beyond doubt that the allegation is true and, if you cannot do that to that level of proof, then we would be seeking to find on behalf of the students. You might wish to say something about that just at this moment because it seems that a big onus is upon you.

A: *My response to that is that there is not so much an onus on me as an onus on the Principle of Invigilation, which is something you have to think about. It is not for me to contemplate the effects of those on other people. Certainly if the invigilator is to be conceptualised as a kind of prosecutor who must convince a jury, then that will certainly have an effect on future invigilation and that is what you have to think about, not me. As for myself, I do not mind. I am not alleging that cheating took place. I am making a statement based upon what I observed. The language of 'alleged' and 'cheating' is not mine. I am merely stating that, as a presiding invigilator, I observed certain events take place and of those observed events there is no doubt and that is that.*

Q: Well, thank you for making your position clear and ours as well. Perhaps we can now move onto the observations that you actually did make on that day. We recognise that this is a serious situation and, therefore, there is a certain degree of formality with that and it is easy to slip into quasi legal definitions, but we do hope that it will be an open discussion and that we will hopefully not be seen here as a prosecuting counsel or as a jury. We do hope to operate by principles of fairness. That is where we would be with that. So maybe if you would just begin wherever you feel easy with about what happened that day in that examination.

A: *I will just quickly look at what I said before…I do not think I have a great deal to add actually. The only thing I could add to the statement I made, which was that approximately 20 minutes before the close of the exam I observed Mr. ******** pass what appeared to be information on his examination paper to Miss ****** and the fact that I said that she appeared to accept and read the information, is that the passing of the paper was blatant. I do not pay a lot of attention myself to non-verbal language, but it was on the level of, 'Have a look at this now and I won't bother to do anything for the next minute or so while you are doing it.' It was so Mickey Mouse obviously blatant that it was* *the only time in 10/12 years of invigilating that there was no doubt in my mind that he was giving her information. It was just obvious on the level that almost reduces it to innocence.*

Q: Perhaps you would say a little bit more abut how blatant that was. You have said you do not pay much account to non-verbal communication, but then you went on to make a number of verbal statements which were interpretations of that. Could you say how it was passed. Was it handed? Was it given? Was it shuffled across?

A: I*t was passed like **that** and he then sat back and looked at the sky and around while she dealt with it as much as to say that he was waiting for her to finish, by which time I was then facing them and he did not make any nervous reaction, he did not act with alacrity; he very deliberately pulled it back as a response to my looking at them. (Indicating) There have been many occasions when I thought that I saw something or perceived or whatever, but I do not act on thoughts, apprehensions or possibilities because I never have had. On this occasion, there was no question in my mind whatsoever, none.*

Mr Mitchell: Can I check one or two things about that. First of all, when you say that he passed it over, was it as deliberate as you are saying there? Was it with his hand not with his elbow?

A: *No, it was with his hand. In fact, I think he actually pointed at the notes he had made for her.*

Q: Whereabouts on the paper?

A: *I do not know.*

Q: As you presented it there, that is one sheet.

A: *Yes.*

Q Can you remember or do you know , was it *that* or was it that? Was the paper open?

A: No, I do not remember.

Q: You do not know whether the paper was open?

A: No, I have no recall. I probably did at the time, but now I do not recall. In fact, immediately at the time I had forgotten that he had actually pointed at something on the paper, I recalled that afterwards.

The Chairman: Is that what you later recovered from the student? [Indicating]

A: Yes, that is right.

Q: Did you ask for that immediately afterwards?

A: I collected those when I collected the scripts, yes.

Q: Having seen the paper, as it were like this, would that refresh your memory any more as to whether he was pointing to this particular page?

A: I would not care to say that, no.

Q: Did you subsequently have a look at any of the papers to see if there were similarities or did you leave that completely to the Board?

A: No, I did not look to see if there were similarities between their written work. I would doubt if there are. There is no doubt in my mind that nothing pre-emptive happened here; it was a moment of madness, perhaps; I do not know. I am not alleging that anything happened; I do not have the faintest idea. I simply saw him pass information.

Q   Which appeared to be accepted from the other candidate?

A: Yes and there does not appear to be anything of a non-examination type on the paper. No, 'kiss, kiss, I love you' mark.

Mr Mitchell: Although the word 'cheating' is used in your second letter.

A: *Only in response to immediate use of language by others, particularly the phrase 'alleged cheating' which I took offence at.*

Q: You took offence at that?

A: *Yes. I have stated from the very beginning that I was the presiding invigilator, I am there in the place of the Board and my decision is final. I am not pushing that angle too far now because I have come against too many obstacles.*

The Chairman: Can you say anything about that.

A: *It was just a personal reaction; I was in the place of the Board; I was presiding invigilator. I mean, who would dream of doing such a thing without there being obvious ground? I never have in the past in all the years when I have thought I have observed things. Only a psychopath would act like this. And a great deal of offence has been taken, not just by me.*

Q: Where has the offence been taken?

A: *That an invigilator's judgement is being questioned, that unless it is a very…Obviously, if someone can ever generate information that the invigilator is the jilted lover of a candidate, then by all means, but there is no connection between me and these students; I hardy know them.I am telling you what I saw and that is that.*

Q: Well, here is another question of judgement. Is there any possibility that alternative interpretations could have been found for that course of action in your judgement?

A: *No.*

Q: It is not something that could have been moved across as the candidate continued to write or shuffled absent-mindedly?

A: *You would have to live in a world where you can take sensibly the question, 'does the table move when you are not in the room?' You would have to live in that kind of world. It was obvious, obvious, obvious.*

Q: If you were to try and move nearer to this world where the table moves, what would be your thoughts on the motivations of the candidates within those circumstance which you observed? What do you think was actually going on there from his position and hers?

A: *A lot of foolishness, I think, I never have regarded this as, if you like, collusion or a serious concerted attempt or anything like that. I believe they have made a lot of play about the fact that he was on one question and she was on another. I mean, what comes to mind is, the police are called to Marks and Spencer and the person is accused of taking something that is worth £1. 80p and they say, 'Why would I do that? I have £100 in my pocket', but they do. Life is like that. I have never suggested that this was anything that was going to benefit them. I do not know. I am simply saying that I saw him pass I mean, I will even take it down to the level of saying that I saw what appeared to be a bluish piece of material. [the examination paper is blue] I will even reduce it to that level if you want because I do not want to allege anything. I am the presiding invigilator and I am obliged to report if I see information being passed from one person to another and I did. If that does not count, then invigilation does not count and the ENB are in a lot of trouble.*

Q: I suppose we see our business as a bit more complicated than that.

A: *OK, yes.*

Q: And in a way not seeking to establish this as some sort of battle in which the ENB loses or wins or the Institute loses or wins.

A: *I am sorry, that is perhaps melodramatic and I perhaps withdraw that. I will leave that side of it to you. I am simply saying that my initial point is a valid one in that I think there is more here than just one person's observation, but what happens, happens.*

Mr Mitchell: Without going on about it too long, even though you do not want to say it or it appears that you do not want to, you must have made an assumption that something irregular happened.

A: *Yes.*

Q: Otherwise there would have been no reason to stop the examination in the afternoon.

A: *Of course, logically you would not have, no.*

Q: So, even though it was not down in black and white, the assumption must have been made somewhere.

A: *Yes, I was absolutely certain of what I had seen, yes, but one has to be very careful about what one says to a body such as this. Nobody wanted to injure them. I mean, professionally we had no difficulty with it, but we certainly did emotionally. Nobody has entered into this with any sense of enthusiasm or anything.*

The Chairman: I would like to just pick up a little bit more on this and we are indeed in grey areas now, but it seems necessary that we try to establish in some ways the motivations of the candidates because that seems to have some impact and some bearing upon what decision we may reach. You have been using words like 'craziness' and 'foolishness' and 'lack of street credibility', words which seem to imply something different than a deliberate attempt to collude and cheat and take advantage of shared information.

A: *I started off and tried very hard to leave it at the behaviourist level. I tried very hard in letter and in word to let it stand at that. It is very difficult because people seem to be* *so concerned as to find out why. I do not know why but, if I am asked often enough, then I will say, 'Well, I do not know; a moment of madness or whatever.' I am not imply-ing anything terrible. Honest to God, I do not know why and, to be perfectly honest with you, I could not give a damn, really.*

Q: Let me just pursue that with you for a moment. Do you think it is a legitimate course of action for us to pursue to try to establish what might be going on for the students?

A: *No, I do not. I believe that, if you have a statement from an Invigilator, if there is contravening evidence or supposi-tions which look promising or in themselves suspicious so as to cast some doubt on that invigilator's decision, then, yes, by all means. I cannot see what that is personally, but that is only my view. It is not for me to....I cannot tell you what to do.*

Mr Mitchell: Can I just come back in to pursue the matter in terms of behaviour or in terms of the incident that oc-curred. Presumably the passing of certain information would not be regarded as being sufficient to report.

A: *I do not know.*

Q: If the person passed a bus time-table—and I know we are getting into silly realms here but I am just trying to check it out—would that be sufficient?

A: *Well, I was speaking to someone the other day about my own school days. We had a teacher who used to tell us to fold our arms and put our head in our arms while he left the room. He did that of course with the great expectation of finding us in the same position when he came back in again and in most cases he did because, when in Rome, you do as the Romans and even as a child there are cer-tain things you know not to do. Why someone would pass a bus time-table to someone while they are doing a final exam, I do not know, nor why they would pass anything. It would seem to me to be a pretty daft thing to do.*

The Chairman: To what extent are these candidates known to you and from your knowledge of them known to each other. Maybe to start with your relationship with these two. You were saying before that you had little knowledge of them.

A: *I have met ***** ****** once or twice in groups of students, ironically helping him prepare for his exams. I have never met *** *** as a teacher; I do not think I have actually taught her or not that I can remember. I met her socially once or twice about three years ago but not in any intimate way. I have no connection with them. As I say, I did have some connection with ******** in terms of preparing the group that he was in for their exams and that is all. He did not stand out in that group as odd or exceptional.*

Q: We are obviously into a potentially very difficult area and I just wanted to say where that is, as it were, for me and that would be, would you have any personal motivation of your own which could have influenced your statements regarding these two students? That is where I am leading.

A: *No. There could be absolutely nothing of any personal nature.*

Q: To what extent would you know of any relationship between the two of them that could tempt them into helping each other with an ordeal like that?

A: *Somebody told me afterwards that they knew each other, but I had not known that. I do not know of anything along those lines. Somebody has said to me that they do know each other, but that would not be surprising. They are not in the same group, but that would mean that they would not know each other as intimately as if they were in the same group. No, I have no knowledge about their relationship.*

Q: I do not think I have any other questions. Maybe there are some things further that you wish to say or to ask or to comment upon.

A: *I do not think so. I think I will leave it. I am happy with the statement I made in writing. The only embellishment on that is just to say that I would not have acted unless I had been sure of what took place. Perhaps an interesting comment, generally, on the nature of nursing in our culture now, if I can just finish by making a remark, which a colleague made, is that from the late seventies and early eighties, we have engendered a culture of everything being relative and acting towards one another as if problems can always be ameliorated—Carl Rogers, his sincerity and genuineness—and it comes as rather a shock when someone turns round and says, 'Hold on a second, that does not work.' It could be said in the culture we have, all the more so because it was me.*

Q: All the more so?

A   *Because it was me. I would have been the last one to be seen as acting in a very interventionist manner, such as that, but there you are. Something was observed.*

Q: Could I just ask you one last thing. What would be a fair outcome in your terms to this situation?

A: *I would like to see both of them deported, obviously! No. I do not really know. I said some weeks ago that I am certainly not looking for blood. There maybe some who are, but I certainly am not. I think a lot of people were actually quite surprised that nothing happened to them. People think, 'Well, in my day, you would have been dismissed instantly and lots of terrible things would have happened to you' and it is something that I suppose has gone round in our minds, I do not know—declaring that attempt null and void. I do not know.*

Q: And that what, there is some evidence of irregularity perhaps?

A: *You see, it cannot possibly be for me to be presumptive enough to make generalisations about it but, at the same time, it is all or nothing, is it not? If people can go into an* *examination which is invigilated and after all the governing body tell us, even though we have continuous assessment, that one must be vigilant Now, it is all or nothing. If people can walk out of the room saying, 'Yes', he says 'I did, but I say I did not', then the system is stupid. I mean, why have it? Why have it? What is the point? If I can come round and say, 'Yes, I know the presiding invigilator says so, but...It is a power relationship; it has nothing to do with right and wrong; it is a power relationship like so much that is in education. It is like a tutor who gives you back a piece of work saying, 'This reads rather vaguely' and it is as crystal clear to you as whatever, but that is it, he is the tutor and, therefore, it is vague and you get on with it. You can make a nonsense of yourself by writing to the Academic Board complaining and all the rest of it and they might change the grade or they might not and you will just make a nonsense of yourself. It is a power relationship. They were caught. I caught them. Having said that, no, I would not want anything dreadful to happen to them. I think that what matters is the principle of whether this is found or not, not what happens to them.*

Q: You do not think that a course of action should follow?

A: *I think that what matters is whether or not you find that what the invigilator stated is correct or not and not the consequences for them afterwards.*

Q: Where does that belong then?

A: *It belongs with you. I do not know what *** ********** would want to do if you decide against them. That is up to her. I would not want anything terrible to happen to them.*

Q: Dismissals and things like that?

A: *No. As I said, I never believed it was a concerted or sustained thing. It was a moment of madness, but....*

Q: It was there. Right, thank you for coming along.

A: *Nice to see you again.*

The Chairman: And you. It is within an awkward setting but that is where we are, is it not, at the moment.

Mrs Storey: Thank you for clearing up the points.

The aftermath

I later had a telephone call from Mr Brown who said that the ENB recognised my integrity, but found in favour of the students. In a follow-up letter, he stated that there was a 'sequence of events that was capable of different interpretation' [and that] 'in view of the lack of substantive and collaborative evidence... the Board decided that the examination attempt should stand.' Clearly, they had little regard for my testimony as substantial. Their decision, they said, was based on the facts of the case with no reflection on my observations and, what's more, they '... respected my integrity.' In future, they would recommend that two invigilators be present [they have] and with all candidates at separate tables. The promised right of appeal was subsequently denied and all requests that they reconsider were denied.

It seemed that, from the outset, the Commission were against the idea of any one truth holding sway: they took the view that there were as many truths as there were people involved. More specifically, the truth, for them, would reside in the meanings, which those involved, attached to events. That being the case, they spent an inordinate amount of time looking into the student's experience of these events and, throughout, they seemed reluctant to come to a judgement. However, one wonders what they might have expected me to do in the circumstances. Whatever the validity of taking different truths at equal value, the fact is the students broke the rules. I made a judgement that two people had committed an infringement: I then judged that it was right to confront them with this and even take it further. The student's instant reaction had been shock that someone had acted against them; that someone had said, 'hold on a second, I want to know what you just did'. These students had been well schooled in the tradition of Rogerian 'theory' and so cannot be fully censured for their response.

At a more general level, Eraut (1994) believes that education systems have moved too far in the direction of experiential methods, probably as a result of anti-intellectualising during the late seventies and eighties. These 'forms of education and the professional competence and expertise they seem to enable, cannot be represented as a publicly accessible knowledge base' (see Bradshaw, 1998: p104). Therefore, what you are left with are educational systems that have, as their core, the idea of the practitioner having sole responsibility for his/her competence: a competence that is not externally measurable, but which derives from experience. Traditionally, education has embraced learning as a two-way process between teacher and learner. This notion of education as a form of exchange is as old as Socrates, whose exchanges with pupils, strangers and enemies are legendary. However, the business of exchange, in and of itself, was never allowed to dislodge truth or accuracy: Socrates would correct the infelicitous comments and barbarisms of his audience. That is what teaching is: responding honestly, having listened very carefully. For many, examinations are the extreme of educational exchange, the moment when candidates must give of their best without assistance other than recall. Many dislike it as a form of assessment: many advocate its abolition. However, on the day in question, it was in position and it symbolised something of the relationship between student and teacher, between learning and a college's responsibility to assess that learning. The two students concerned abused that right and I rightfully judged them for it. It's a paradox that, if the commission members truly believed that 'each person represents a truth', then they could have found equally in favour of me or them. This is why perhaps they were keen to vouchsafe my veracity. However, there remained the awkward facts of the case and, on this occasion, they came to a dual conclusion: I was awarded integrity and the students were given 'the decision'.

As for invigilators today, what to do if they witness an infringement of the rules? My advice would be look away.

5
The veracity of scientific nursing

Preamble

From its religious beginnings to its present incarnation as a physical science, it would be nice to think that psychiatry's development had followed a natural progression. Such progressions are rare however so that, for instance, the apparent 'triumph' of psychoanalysis in the 1930s, arguably its heyday, in Britain at any rate, eventually yields to its current demise. Equally, the mindless psychiatry of the 1940s and 1950s—exemplified by the physical treatments approach of William Sargant (1967)—went hand-in-hand with the supposed benefits of social psychiatry (Jones 1952). It is fascinating to recall that as R.D. Laing (1961) postulated a philosophical psychiatry (co-opting, in the process, the 'madman' as brother-philosopher), William Sargant was describing himself as 'a physician in the practice of psychological medicine'.

Thus, the central division that has existed in psychiatry since its foundation is between a medical practice, based on scientific principles, that seeks to unearth the physical causes of mental disease, as opposed to a non-medical group that sees mental illness as a 'different way of being' and tries to address the experiences and needs of those affected.

Without question, the medical approach has come to personify psychiatric practice in Britain and Europe. However, it has achieved this at the cost of being characterised (by the non-medical group) as too detached—even heartless—in its application. Also, for all of the alleged accomplishments of medical psychiatry, the beliefs of the non-medical group remain as strong as ever. Medical aficionados would probably say that such non-scientific views are simply an irrelevance, a bad hangover from the 1960s with its wildly speculative philosophies and radical-chic ideas.

Nurses

Looking at how nurses fit into this division, no better description exists than Dave Pilgrim's (1983) depiction of them as 'fellow travellers'. Classically, most psychiatric nurses have followed the medical lead in respect of diagnosis and physical treatments of patients. Few question these treatments, or their so-called side-effects: historically, nurse commentators can be seen to advocate such treatments, both covertly (Stein 1978) and openly (Gray 1998).

Having said that, non-medical nursing also has its followers. Although smaller in number, these nurses remain broadly sceptical of the claims of brain sciences to ultimately cure mental disorder. Although as knowledgeable—as knowledgeable as nurses can be—of the complexities of molecular brain sciences, non-medical nurses insist on retaining a philosophical inquiry—drawing from social and psychological research—into the meaning of mental illness, especially the question of how nurses should respond to it.

It is ironic that although psychiatrists can entertain a variety of notions on the nature of mental illness—the second largest interest group in the Royal College of Psychiatrists is its philosophy section—a group of psychiatric nurses continue to vigorously campaign for biological explanations. Because of the abrasive tone brought to debate by this group, and their refusal to discuss many of the issues involved, as well as their evident disdain for philosophising about these issues, I came to characterise them as the new nurse brutalists (Clarke, 1999c). A harsh term, perhaps, but deserved on several grounds. Firstly, because their characterisation of non-medical groups as 'woolly and out-dated', was likely to bring nursing into intellectual disrepute. Secondly, through their position as a spearhead movement that seems to merge scientific, commercial, and corporate interests into, what Dwight Fee (2000: p5) calls', a new technocratic system of inert diagnostics'. Within such systems, the patient's narrative is at risk of being lost.

New century

Charles Golden and Jana Sawicki (1985) typify those who believe that science will ultimately unravel 'the latent secrets of diseased minds'. Convinced that 'neurological approaches provide effective methods of investigating psychopathological disorders', they believe that 'such approaches will be among the major contributions of the twentieth and twenty-first centuries'. Well, pardon me, but did I miss something? Surely such a lauded science would, by now, have provided us with more than a cache of over-priced anti-psychotic drugs, a brain machine that shocks people out of depression, as well as a group of less potent, but highly addictive pills for camouflaging anxiety and alienation? Yet, despite the fact that little in real terms has actually happened, a new optimism in the brain sciences persists. According to Nesse and Williams (1995), neuro-pharmacological research 'spurred on by drug companies has re-created sharp distinctions between symptom clusters as opposed to psychological factors'. In addition, these findings have produced exaggerated claims that humankind is now on the brink of solving its most intractable and complex mental problems, perhaps even schizophrenia itself. Not for nothing have we been 'exhorted to re-badge mental illnesses as brain illnesses' (Burns, 2000), as though this was the only way of seeing psychological distress.

Steven Rose (1998) points out that current fascination with genetics and technology has not struck quite the same virulent tone in Britain as in America, but notes, nevertheless, that 'the number of academic journals with some permutation of the words neuro, brain and behaviour is now running into the hundreds'. Doubtless, many would like to restrict discussions to this level and in some cases rightly so. However, in Great Britain, the brutalist element is keen to stress the central role of molecules, genes, transmitter substances and neurological cavities in the aetiology of functional mental illness as well. For these nurses, mental illness requires a scientific rationale, as well as a grounding in (what is now called) evidence-based practice. These nurses have a low tolerance for what they regard as the post-sixties, post-modern, post-

Laingian confabulations of an anti-psychiatric brigade that obstinately refuses to acknowledge the 'breathtaking achievements' of modern day science.

Is science sufficient?

Scientific approaches are an insufficient basis upon which to discuss mental illness, if we include the perspective of individual experience. For this perspective, we need to introduce constructs, such as anxiety, memory, attitude, fear, and loathing. These constructs fit more plausibly within a concept of mind rather than brain, not just because of the absence of any anatomical explanations for them, but more so because 'mind' accommodates the hypothetical nature of these constructs, as well as their diverse meanings for different people. It is in this sense that removing from a philosophical inquiry of mind, those experiences, defined by psychiatry as ill, seems oddly arbitrary. It is a curious philosophical twist that assumes some human thought can be the province of medical speculation because medicine defines that thought as ill.

In many ways, the body/mind question is (in psychiatric terms) neurological science's last frontier in that establishing a physical cause for schizophrenia, for example, would represent a significant advance of matter over mind. This seems improbable, however, as it is mind that encompasses subjectivity—the acquisition of life experiences. Obviously, any talk of mind as a separate entity must be repugnant to anyone committed to chemical-electrical explanations of behaviour. Thankfully, this kind of scientism may be on the wane and recent mind/brain texts (Glynn, 1999; Kohn, 1999; Midgley, 2001) seem less keen to assert fixed-entity neuro-properties as explanations for behaviour. Although many psychiatrists remain open-minded, as noted, some nurses continue to pursue more hard-wired descriptions of behaviour and with a peculiar inclination to react positively to whatever 'new findings' come their way.

The kingdom is nigh

It pays to be on one's guard against 'imminent breakthrough' rhetoric. Something that the recent explosion of brain/mind books brought in its wake was an 'inexorable drive of science' verbosity. In some nursing circles, a kind of swagger entered debate and an 'on the brink', 'we may confidently expect', type of thinking mushroomed. Although advances in the physical treatment of psychiatric patients remained erratically slow, belief in the organic basis of, what now came to be called, 'serious and enduring mental illness' continued to grow. Not that the protagonists of this had everything their own way.

Challenges to biological psychiatry proceeded apace along several fronts. Boyle (1990), for instance, identified some illogical assumptions inherent in schizophrenic diagnoses. Barker (1997) resolutely defended the role of individual experience in understanding psychiatric distress and Clarke (1999c) detected an ideological bias in much of what tried to pass in nursing literature as scientific inquiry. The persistence of these challenges vexed, but rarely hampered those bent on locating mental illness within biological and/or genetic frameworks. Buoyed up by the belief that 'their time had come', neurological visionaries embraced a habitat of genes for sorrow, genes for joy, fecklessness, aggression, suicide, and sadism. Daniel Koshland, editor of the journal *Science*, postulated a gene for homelessness and the London Observer (2000) reported a gene that predisposed people to commit suicide. At present, a research team at London's University College Medical School is examining the history of aversion therapy in relation to gay people, partly as 'a timely reminder of the interplay between science and society in an era of rapid discoveries within biological and medical sciences'. In America, such 'reparative therapy', although condemned by the American Psychiatric Association, is on the move again. Nobody expects that we are about to re-invent 'reparative therapy' in Britain, but, as Robert Munro (2001) points out, the problem lies in the 'the attraction of giving those who do not conform to one's own view of morality a spurious psychiatric diagnosis.' Equally, the Faustian credibility of 'genetics' gives comfort to anyone intending to ignore the wishes of those who might be affected by medical diagnoses. What, for example, would be the moral implications of a gene for suicide or for Alzheimer's? Would employers, for instance, be entitled to require employees or applicants to take tests, which might indicate their possession of the gene and, thus, their long-term fitness or economic viability?

Of course, a lot of what we do in life is a product of genetic inheritance. Most of us accept that human beings are a product of nature **and** nurture. However, it is the relative weight that we attach to one or the other of these, which has proved contentious. While postulating specific genetic pathways for identifiable human behaviours is possible—it is done, for example, in the case of phenylketonuria or Huntington's Chorea—making similar claims in respect of schizophrenia is more problematic. This is not because it is true, but, instead, because the scientific nature of its (part) truth and the diagnostic dimension that it invokes can have the effect of minimising or even trivialising approaches that put the experiences of those affected first. Few would deny the existence of a genetic component in schizophrenia, but its mode of transmission is nowhere as clear as something like Huntington's. Nor could such genetic information about schizophrenia be presently utilised in treatment programmes, other than as a crude indicator for pregnancy terminations. However, the point for nurses is about how such information is used, how it fits within the narrative exchanges between nurse and patient.

Medical diffidence

Interestingly, the medical profession has affected a greater scepticism towards the new biotechnology. For instance, Anthony Clare (1999), while acknowledging the contribution of molecular genetics and PET scan technology, wondered if these developments represented a 'reincarnated neuro-psychiatry'. Quoting Leon Eisenberg (1997) that in the USA 'a rampant biological psychiatry' had emerged as an outcome of managerial pressure, Clare cautioned against drawing conclusions from inconclusive evidence, and was rather cool about current efforts to dispense with a social psychiatric culture built up over the last 200 years. In London, Professor of Community Psychiatry, Tom Burns (2000), similarly warns against conceptualising mental illness as brain dysfunction: 'personally, I don't think that mental illnesses happen in the brain or in the synapses between brain cells. Whilst brain dysfunction may be relevant, mental illnesses happen between people, or between an individual and his own inner representation' (p166). The last line could so easily have been written by the 1960s radical psychiatrist RD Laing and coming from the pen of an orthodox practitioner, is an indication of how timeless some of Laing's ideas are.

Yet within psychiatric nursing, some remain determined to embrace neuropsychiatry. Martin (1999b), for example, sets herself the task of educating nurses about 'brain changes' in depressed people. 'Significant reductions in cerebral blood flow in specific areas of the frontal lobe and limbic systems occur', she says, 'because these areas of the brain are switched off during episodes of major depression. Antidepressant therapy', she goes on, 'switches these areas back on'. Hardly surprising when you consider that by antidepressant therapy she means electric treatment. Other approaches likely to switch patients back on, she states, are drugs, cognitive therapy, total sleep deprivation and something called interpersonal psychotherapy (IPT). The latter sets out to give the patient a 'sick role' and thus diminish personal guilt and responsibility for whatever 'condition' they may have. Practitioners of IPT, for example, will show patients copies of their brain scan pictures, presumably so that they can see that their experience of depression is not 'them'.

Curiously enough, advocates of neurological nursing are often unable to forgo the personal in discussions about their clients. Martin's description of IPT fails to see the contradiction between her proposed neurological framework, its visual representation in PET scan machines and the experiences of her patients. Ironically, given her neurological perspective, she lists the likely causes of her patient's distress as a) complicated bereavement; b) role dispute; c) role transition; and d) interpersonal factors. In my view, all of these are compounded of psychological, spiritual, and social factors and the annoying thing is not the legitimacy of using physical methods to treat them, but the excessive homage ascribed to physical treatments, almost as if they possessed antidote status.

Nevertheless, recent years have seen modest increases in factual descriptions of mental illness and no doubt neuro-biologists will continue to distinguish the abnormal from the normal human brain. Ultimately, they may demonstrate positive correlations between certain forms of behaviour and neural blood flow, oxygen uptake, and the like. What they cannot show is why some behaviours are seen as abnormal to begin with. Apart from the fact that existing studies do not show a close correspondence between abnormal brains and psychiatric syndromes (Kitwood, 1988), it is a questionable exercise that construes abnormal behaviour without some regard for morality, culture, and history. In the final analysis, of course, brain studies will never account for personal experience: possibly they might in another three to four thousand years. This, however, hardly matters to nurses now, or to their patients.

Natural born theories

Why does this movement to reinvent a biological psychiatry exist? Bold rather than courageous, these nurses are intent on transforming psychiatric nursing from a humanistic endeavour to a cognitivist-behaviourist 'science'. Driven by a sulphuric belief in the biological basis of behaviour, as well as an enduring faith in the ability of medical science to 'deliver', they insist that empiricism, in the form of randomised controlled trials and 'collaborative research with medicine', is the only way by which psychiatric nursing can advance.

Predictably, these nursing brutalists are aggressive; theirs is a scientism that does 'not suffer fools gladly'. Not for them the pusillanimous vagaries of person-centred nurse theorists: not for them the uncomfortableness of research paradigms that obstinately retain experience as an important consideration of what constitutes mental illness. Indeed, it is the attachment to experience and its narrative outcomes that particularly annoys the brutalists who, when not counting numbers, prefer a clipped, topped, and tailed (if somewhat forced) style of writing. Susan Ritter (1997), for one, often uses the trick of beginning verbal and written 'statements' with the same phrase couched in interrogative form: 'We need to ask this, we need to ask that, we need to ask the other... ' and so on. In an interesting passage (p99), she begins five successive sentences with 'Apart from behaviour therapy... ' each sentence including an important function of which non-behaviourists are deemed incapable. That behaviour therapy evolved within clinical psychology (only to be subsequently 'borrowed' by nurses under the leadership of a psychiatrist, Isaac Marks), seems not to faze her. Certainly, if the intention is to define nursing as behaviourism, then this hardly says much about what is unique to nursing. Not that this is an important consideration of this group: theirs is an altogether more ambitious task, involving a virtual re-definition of the nursing role as a quasi-medical enterprise. That task stems in part from an extraordinary attachment to randomised control trials (RCTs), and they seem peculiarly unable to see these as anything more than one method of accruing particularised forms of knowledge. Rather is there a trumpeting of these trials as the 'gold standard' of research. Nurses are encouraged to embrace this approach rather than, for example, qualitative research that is seen as 'soft' or anecdotal. In my view, this emphasis on RCTs is mistaken, and I propose to say why. As a first principle, subjects in RCTs should represent the target population to which any trial results will apply. As such, to generalise from results obtained from two sets of diagnosed subjects from within, let's say, two community health teams, when others with the same diagnosis (of schizophrenia) continue to inhabit hospital populations is misleading. The life histories of people described as schizophrenic, as well as their current social status, is an important consideration in constructing research programmes with them as subjects.

Further, how does one ensure randomisation when investigating people with schizophrenia, where informed consent may be difficult to obtain? Investigations into groups whose rationality is questionable—in terms of the investigators own definitions—leads to difficulties in obtaining informed consent. Of course, it is the heterogeneity of schizophrenia that is the issue here: baffling differences exist between people with schizophrenia—it is essentially a subjective 'condition'—and only by ignoring these differences can the virtues of RCTs be asserted. Indeed, given the desirability of having large sample sizes in randomised trials, the sample sizes typically employed by psychiatric nurse researchers (to date) have rarely satisfied these requirements. And, even if 'representative' numbers of subjects are obtained, this confounds matters all the more given the noted heterogeneity of the 'condition'. In fact, this becomes an instance in which numerical 'more' means theoretical 'less'. The point is that matching subjects from different (experimental and control) groups is going to be difficult because such matching procedures:

> *are predicated on the assumption that diseases have common features which can be identified, quantified, analysed and communicated. Yet not only is diagnosing and defining disease notoriously difficult, but its passage is not predictable or consistent within any pathology.'*

(Hicks, 1998: p26)

In the light of this, how do you assess the worth of an individual's verbal statements: how do you operationally define a psychotic individual's delusions? And, in any event, would nurses particularly want to? The truth is that nurse-patient interventions do not lend themselves to the reductionist parameters of RCTs: to boot, such trials violate the person-centred principles to which (some) nursing currently aspires.

The necessity of RCTs for determining the viability of drugs and other physical treatments is unanswerable. It would be unthinkable to market a drug that had not been tested using double-blind, randomised methods. The question for nurses, however, is whether the conditions which constitute nursing can be 'reduced' to the levels of controllability that would withstand quantitative investigation. Or are there aspects of nurse-patient relationships that are not conducive to RCTs? If so, does it follow that these aspects are trivial or peripheral? How you answer that will say a good deal about the kind of nurse you are.

I suspect that the rigour attending RCTs in areas, such as pharmacology, is not possible in 'social' research and, while this is fair enough, it would help if nurse researchers occasionally acknowledged it. The point is that if any comparable difficulties, of the kind described here, were to occur in a RCT in pharmacology, it would be discontinued.

Really, RCTs in nursing have, at best, a static, 'emptied out' feel to them, lacking any connection with their subject's experiences. Rather are these RCTs connected to policy and management dimensions of people living in 'the community' and often with a 'what best to do about them' element built in. To that end, such trials have increased in recent years, possibly as a consequence of the need for purchasers and providers of health care to have something upon which to base their decisions. It is a sad fact that qualitative studies tend to be rejected by funding organisations in preference to studies that demonstrate evidence-based outcomes, usually linked to probable policy initiatives. Research does not take place in a vacuum and political requirements are not easily separated from the motivations of nurse (or other) researchers.

In a study of relationships within a nursing unit, Clarke and Cornish (1972) learned the hard way that quantitative methods did not easily encompass the complex vagaries of their subject matter. In order to work, they concluded, a RCT has to pair one set of interventions against another so as to establish which is 'better' in respect of the problem being considered. Such 'winner takes all' research is all very well—as drug companies know to their advantage—but, outside of physical medicine, it fails to account for the multiple factors, particularly where there are competing psychosocial interventions under review, which contribute to how one approach becomes preferable over another. Unless one knows **that**, unless one knows what confers superiority to one approach over another, then findings cannot be generalised. This is the central problem for RCTs in a nursing context. Where human relationships are contributory elements in treatment or care programmes, it becomes difficult for RCTs to assess their effects. This is because of the difficulty of linking human experience to other items that emerge in the research in any causally unambiguous way. For RCTs to become plausible within nursing contexts, they would need to be able to specify the nursing contribution in the form of itemised interventions; in other words they would have to fit the 'nursing' to the research. This can be a difficult thing to do, especially when elements of value judgement or attitudinal factors are involved. In Caroline Hick's view (1998: p23), 'the interaction between patient and carer is beyond the scope of RCT evaluation'. It is **interaction** that is seen as comprising the nursing contribution. Having said this, not all interactions between people are of an emotional or reflective nature. A nurse who practices behaviour therapy, for example, might insist that her interventions are distinct and measurable as against no interventions at all. It might be possible that a limited form of controlled trial could take account of different types of psychological interventions and be in a position to draw broad conclusions. Such a wide-angled approach would not match the specificity of drug trials, or orthodox scientific research generally. More importantly, it would require nursing to redefine itself as a form of psychological therapy and this would be at odds with traditional concepts of nursing where, essentially, it is distinguished from therapy.

Motivation

Professor Kevin Gournay is perhaps the chief protagonist of RCTs. With like-minded colleagues (Wray, 1994; Bennett *et al*, 1995; Gournay and Ritter, 1997; Gournay *et al*, 1997; Gray, 1998; Brooker and Repper, 1998) he would have us believe that they are scientists, devotees of the laboratory bench. He says it himself: 'schizophrenia is genetic, depression is genetic, the "medical model" works' (Gournay, 1998: p41). Of course, the truth, as I've said, is that we are all genetic and what is to be gained by naming schizophrenic patients as such is hard to fathom. True, genetic research may one day prevent the occurrence of some mental illnesses, but what is the relevance of that to nurses working with patients now? We do well, instead, to look at ways in which science is applied to human groups. Malevolence has never been so horridly effective than when cloaked in the white-coated respectability of scientific advance and scientific justification. In the light of this, it would fare nurses better to protect patients from the excesses of scientific applications rather than rushing pell-mell to embrace 'new discoveries', which may mean little in the practical lives of people. What seems lacking in the nursing brutalists is any appreciation of this; of the need to understand science within contexts. How easily we forget bad science, ugly science—the crude genetics of the 1930s, for instance. 'Oh, I'm sorry, pardon me: it wasn't the science that was bad', you say, 'it was the way that it was used'. Well, exactly, and this is why naively picking up on some modest advances in medical technology—scan readings of ventricle enlargements and enhanced blood flow—and using these as clarion calls for new forms of 'assertive' nursing is so very misguided.

'I have sat in the scanning room and watched people's brains lighting up as they hallucinate in a way that normal brains don't.'

(Gournay, 1998: p41)

Whether through tongue in cheek or blind faith, the effect of statements like these is to belittle discussion, to diminish whatever experience may lie behind the virtual realities of the TV monitor. It is important that nurses do not fall into the trap of ignoring personal heartache by only dealing with suffering that sports a policy dimension. Of course, everyday experience is difficult to gauge in formal terms; it is hardly the stuff of which 'scientific' reports are made. Nevertheless, one expects nurses to attend to experience: to respect the 'rightness' of other people's perceptions of their problems. What jars, as such, is the spectacle of nurses—**nurses**—doing policy makers' work for them: effectively disenfranchising people whose psychological problems are seen as undeserving of psychiatric nursing interventions because they are not 'serious and enduring'. In effect, these nurses constitute a fifth column operating on behalf of medical concepts, seeking to consolidate these within psychiatric nursing practice.

Probably, the most transparent example of this was the 1994 paper by Gournay and Brooking, which used a RCT approach to examine therapeutic effectiveness among groups of community psychiatric nurses. In an incisive review of this paper, Tilley and Ryan (2000) showed how these writers 'linked CPNs to psychiatry by case loads or by specialist technique and legitimated these links by reference to literature, which indicated they were effective whilst drawing from (other) literature which indicated that CPNs not so linked were not effective.' Of course, in doing this, you could say that Gournay and Brooking were simply playing the game of garnering literature in support of their pre-determined views. However, the difficulty, in their case, is that they purport to represent an evidenced-based view, a view that originates from the science bench, and forms the 'gold standard' of RCTs. In their study, Gournay and Brooking tried to show that the 'counsellor nurse' was ineffective, but, to achieve this, as Tilley and Ryan show, they had to resort to formulating 'counsellor-nurses' as a 'scandal', as a 'squandering of resources' and an 'abandonment' of the severely mentally ill'.

In my preamble, I mentioned the distaste that the medical group exhibit towards philosophising of any kind, even to the point of ignoring important criticisms of their views. Well, in respect of the paper by Tilley and Ryan (2000), for instance, Professor Gournay (2000), invited to respond, simply reproduced an updated version of the rhetoric that had warranted the Tilley and Ryan critique in the first place. Such dismissals are the downside of an overbearing confidence, which takes as read that people from opposite or different camps are living 'in the past', unable to see that what counts, nowadays, is the utility of information, concepts that are serviceable, cost effective and unsullied by the messiness of human experience. Miller Mair (1989: p32), drawing from Godzich (1984), states that:

> 'information is not so much stored to be reflected upon as it is consumed. Instead of contributing to the growing awareness of the person's continuity with others in space and time it breaks up time and space, isolates the person from others, and unmoors

him or her by subjecting everything to the momentary needs of the market'.

In this case, it is the control over research funding that invalidates human experience as a form of inquiry. Education curricula that does likewise severs personal experience as a 'developed means of knowing', so that students end up acclimatised only to what is or is not marketable as professional activity.

Never mind the quantity, feel the depth

In trying to understand 'sick' people, it is important to attend to their experiences and to do that, naturally, is a qualitative exercise. Pointing an accusative finger at the failure of qualitative research to live up to 'the gold standard' of RCTs is missing the point. It is a bit like asking qualitative methods to account for double-blind drug trials. Equally, it is absurd to address issues of human experience in a statistical, detached manner. It is not that quantitative approaches, for example, questionnaires, are incapable of extracting **some** information of a personal and relevant nature from psychiatrically ill subjects, but, in terms of how people may be experiencing illness, some approach that will recognise the validity of their narrative seems needed.

These are not questions of 'either/or': one accepts the appropriateness of different approaches to different research questions. However, it is important to reject postures that evince little irony in their condemnation of qualitative research, research that, at the end of the day, is but an extension of human communication. In his essay, 'The Nonsense of Effectiveness' (1998), Don Bannister stated that, were we to ask how effective conversation is, we would need to begin by questioning the question. Given the many possible meanings of 'effective', it becomes nonsense just to ask it. And, if we allow a resemblance between conversation and psychotherapy, it seems equally foolish how this self-same question is repeatedly asked of psychotherapists, the intention being, of course, to show how 'ineffective' it all is. For Bannister, morality is not so much about establishing the benefits of therapy, rather it is about paying heed to the narratives of those involved. Further, 'one does this because one's experience of doing therapy makes sense, it is validated in the way of doing it and it is intuitively right, *whatever the literature may say*' (Bannister's italics). This point approximately fits my contention that nursing, by its nature, entails a moral obligation to respond to people, even in the absence of a so-called evidence-base or 'proven' techniques. In some instances, to be with people while they experience distress becomes the essence of the undertaking.

The knowledge base

Part of the problem for nurses is that, in doing research, they find themselves caught up in the philosophical tradition of splitting off sense perception from thinking so that, in keeping with the development of physical sciences, quantitative inquiries are made to appear more conventionally 'proper'. However, one way of over-valuing quantitative approaches is to confuse methods that justify or replicate knowledge (i.e., methods that give us less cause to question things) with issues, which are to do with the sources of knowledge. This difference, between the origins of knowledge and the procedures by which knowledge is verified, is a distinction too often overlooked. As far as nurses are concerned, it may be of less importance to examine principles of verification and more relevant to value knowledge in terms of its origins between people. We commonly respond to theoretical assertions with the demand: 'What is your evidence for that?' And it's a fair question, because, if a theory is about something—even another theory—then there ought to be something about the other theory that shows the main theory to be true (or not). However, while such considerations engender doubt about the nature of verbal reports (on their own) as evidence, this is a pity because it is not as 'evidence' that such reports evolve. Rather they evolve in relationships where two or more people struggle to make sense of their situation. We must live with the inherent subjectivity of exchanged meanings as necessarily incompatible with quantification. There is actually something distasteful about subjecting exchanged meanings to quantitative analysis. Of course, in our society, particular forms of knowledge count more than others: to say that something is 'not scientific' is, these days, to say something vaguely dismissive about it. In fact, most of us recognise that the physical sciences can provide proof to a level of validity that outstrips anything the humanistic 'sciences' have to offer. The issue, however, is the relationship between the two types of knowledge, and their relevance to psychiatric nursing. The question is about the extent to which the narratives of those affected by mental disturbance should play a part in constructing solutions to the problems, which that disturbance brings. This is not to edge out medical relevance, but to place it at the disposal of mentally ill people, to see it as one element among several, which might prove useful to their well-being and not as something that deciphers human nature to the point where relationships are neglected.

Serious and enduring

If the nursing brutalists have nailed their colours to a mast, it has to be the RCT. However, a close second in their pecking order of importance must be 'serious and enduring mental illness'. Like their attempts at RCTs, it is a crude undertaking to put it mildly. On the question of seriousness in mental illness, for example, who defines it? Few would deny that schizophrenia and manic depression are 'serious', but they hardly exhaust seriousness. In defining seriousness, what happens if disagreements emerge? What, for example, counts as non-serious and what if those who are designated 'non-serious', seriously disagree with their non-serious diagnosis? What distinguishes the non-serious from malingering? Or is there some implication that little, indeed, does separate them?

Witness an imaginary BBC News announcement: 'Mr. Wellbeloved had been turned away by St Swithin's on the grounds of not being ill enough: the hospital has since apologised to his family saying that Mr. Wellbeloved's suicide was entirely regrettable. The hospital vigorously deny that Mr. Wellbeloved was told that he had not been ill for long enough.

It was more a case, said a hospital apologist, of his illness lacking an element of seriousness. However, said the same hospital spokesperson, consideration is now being given to the introduction of a Register of Seriousness, in addition to which a Committee of Inquiry has recommended the establishment of a 'Multi-Phasic Indicator of Seriousness Scale': special training programmes in the use of these scales are to be immediately implemented'.

That the Mental Health Nursing Review Team (1994) made an (oft quoted) recommendation in favour of tackling the needs of 'seriously mentally ill people' is neither here nor there, given its neglect of what these terms might actually mean. Here is what they might mean.

> *'Her peace of mind was not deeply disturbed; but she felt sad and once even burst into tears, though she could not have said why…She had a feeling of guilt. The pressure of various vague emotions—the sense of life passing by, a longing for novelty—had forced her to a certain limit, forced her to look behind her, and there she had seen not even an abyss, but only a void…chaos without shape.'*

(p126)

This is Turgenev's (1965; ed) description of Madame Odintsov and it has a corrosive edge to it: when thoughts like these persist, they drain the life (or the death) out of you. Against a background of loss, unexpected bereavement especially, such thoughts lead to desolation. Identifying such predicaments as unworthy of attention, as invalid forms of suffering is, in the context of nursing, genuinely shocking. The Jewish theologian Martin Buber (1970) said, 'Through the Thou, A Man becomes I'. That is to say, to the extent that I treat you with decency, I obtain decency. This is, at least in principle, part of the 'what' of nursing. In other words, there exists a moral obligation to respond to suffering and this holds true, even in the absence of effective techniques or guarantees of outcome. It simply is not good enough to suppose that, like battery hens, psychiatric nurses will be 'licensed to treat' via 'Thorn Initiatives' and other pre-packaged programmes. Such programmes are not 'the best we have got': they are perhaps a worthwhile therapeutic tool (in a long line of such tools) albeit, in reality, no more than a re-packaging of what many nurses do anyway. That 're-packaging' is, of course, an important means by which a professional group may 'improve' its position. The 'best that we have got', that **nurses** have got, is the determination to be vigilant about how therapeutic programmes are used, to remain sceptical of practitioners who seek to objectify patients at the expense of their declared wants.

Moving on

A recent development in this debate has been for some commentators (Burnard and Hannigan, 2000; Repper, 2000) to step back, reflect, and then announce that they are going to present a more objective analysis. This objectivity usually finds its spot precariously balanced on the nearest conceptual fence to hand. In Repper's (2000) opinion, for example, 'an objective mental health nursing base' is improbable and so we need to 'embrace diversity within the practice, research, and explanatory theories of our profession' (p585). Patients, she says, are uninterested in theories and the nursing profession could best move on by leaving aside blanket condemnations or assertions of certainty. While, on the face of it, sounding sensible enough, part of the difficulty with this is that people **do** possess genuinely differing beliefs about psychiatric practice, its effects on people, and its political functions within any given society. Of course, such differing beliefs are only half of a more general equation. People invest a great deal of emotion in what they assert about psychiatry and its application to patients. It was Niechtze who said that, ultimately, 'all argument represents a desire of the heart'. The issue is not about blanket condemnations of other people's certainties, but rather an evaluation of those certainties in terms of their propensity to inflict oppressive therapies on unwilling patients. Of course, this is as much an emotional as an intellectual terrain. In this respect, I differ from Professor Phil Barker (2000) who, responding to Repper, said that different 'world views' are no better than each other, simply different.

I believe that nonconformist elements in psychiatric nursing are of greater benefit, ultimately, to patients because, without this dimension, patients will be subjected to untrammelled medical intrusion and at the expense of their experiences and desires. It is often the case that nonconformists **sound** rasping and over-state their case. This, however, is what being a minority entails: when the funding (for research) goes elsewhere, when it is the medical group which invariably chairs government committees and sundry advisory panels, how can anyone evince surprise if more primitive voices draw attention to the capacity of psychiatry (still) to diminish people and not enhance them.

Institutionalised

Nursing has 'existed' for a thousand years, and 'owning up' to this places one, historically and culturally, in a different position to other related disciplines. It is this moral dimension that the brutalists fail to address. If Don Bannister is right that most responses to people in distress are institutionalised, then no group epitomises this responding more than psychiatric nurses. As we speak, Orwell himself wouldn't half be pleased with nursing: pleased with the professionalism, the easy acceptance of forensic incarceration, the happy embrace of the techniques of 'control and restraint', the abysmal absence of irony at the sinister language of 'assertive outreach'. The benightedness that refuses to accept the complexities, conscious or otherwise, which lead some patients to decline treatments; the accompanying denial that civil liberties may be violated when compulsorily 'treating' patients in 'the community' are all typical of much modern discourse. To the 'science' that would objectify human behaviour so as to control, measure, and treat it as abnormal; to those who would turn their backs on experience as the central healing ground of distress, I would respond by paraphrasing two of my heroes: the Rev Ian Kyle Paisley and the Blessed Margaret of Grantham: No! No! No!

6
See no evil, hear no evil

Irish beginnings

My first exposure to institutionalised violence occurred many years ago, more than thirty to be exact, and before I emigrated to England. It came about while training to be a nurse in a hospital in Southern Ireland for what were then called mentally handicapped people. An enclosed community of male patients with profound learning difficulties and a nursing staff under pressure to keep them 'well behaved' had somehow fostered a climate in which corporal punishment, usually of an instinctive, if in some cases intentionally benevolent, kind had taken hold. At the same time, another kind of punishment, more deliberate, more brutal, also prevailed, although to a lesser extent in the sense of being perpetrated by fewer people.

That those on the receiving end of these punishments were incapable of knowing why they were being beaten seemed not to deter the punishers in the slightest. I suppose, being Irish, we were used to it: most of us had been brought up on it and, although Ireland would be amongst the first to bend to European Union pressure and abolish corporal punishment, at the time, many parents and teachers saw it as an indispensable tool of child rearing. At my primary school, in the 1950s, the implement of discipline was the bamboo cane: one teacher's nickname derived from his committed and zealous use of it. The derivation of his nickname—'skidger'— came from the skid marks left on the palms by the contact of bamboo and flesh. This was a culture of retribution and violence.

Whereas in England

The pressures on nurses within the large mental handicap communes—called colonies in Britain—were very great, not just because of the large numbers of patients they contained and the lack of facilities, but also because of beliefs about the propensity of the patients for unruliness and even violence. Such beliefs, and the repressive practices to which they gave rise, frequently induced, in the staff, a general malaise coupled with a sense of abandonment. For the nurse-attendants, the suspicion that they were carrying out society's 'dirty work' was rarely far from their minds. Although the conditions of care might fluctuate—during World War II staffing levels were particularly low, the ever increasing numbers of people trying to cope with progressively deteriorating asylum conditions became a scandal that was increasingly difficult to contain. At the same time, what continued to matter to the asylum administrators—what had always mattered to them—was order, discipline, and the good behaviour of both the patients and their keepers. An air of Victorian rectitude pervaded these institutions and, for many staff, this fostered a belief that they should be grateful for their occupational role within them. This was partly because these institutions were seen as having moral authority. The gratitude factor—and many were grateful—went hand-in-hand with the immigrant status of many of the nurses who, as a consequence of this, were doubly aware of the need to obey orders without quibble. Since loss of job entailed a loss of practically everything (including, for example, residency permits), immigrants were in no position to question asylum/hospital systems whose constituent (and facilitative) functionaries they became. For most of us, at the time, any capacity to perceive that things might be wrong gave way to a resigned acceptance of things being as they were because that was what the system required. When a government committee (DHSS, 1971) inquired into abuses at Farleigh hospital, for example, they found that 'the standards by which the hospital were judged were its own internal standards' (p7). The Inquiry also discovered that anyone questioning those standards was simply laughed at.

It is difficult to describe how demoralised nurses were within the asylums during the 1950s and onwards. Part of the problem is that institutionalisation diminishes the human capacity to express feelings or beliefs and there exists an apprehension that such expressions will be viewed as tanta-mount to anarchy. One learned fast that mechanistic responses worked best. Working in such conditions made it difficult to identify the processes that sustained these prac-tices.

An enlightened administration—and there were a few—might find itself confronting a nursing staff who, paradoxi-cally fearing and mistrusting their superiors, would ada-mantly reject change in favour of the status quo. What typi-cally happened was that we progressed from being demoralised to a state of complacency and, in some cases, a certain comfortableness with our roles. Of course, there may well have been many who did experience turmoil, but how can one know? It was hardly an age of 'sharing feelings'; in truth, any expression of emotion or reluctance to service the institution's needs would have been regarded as distinctly odd. Nurse education, until the late 1970s, was very much a training allied to medicine, with students ultimately responsi-ble to hospital managers. There was little that was theory-led or that could even be discussed outside the constraints of hos-pital mandates or policies. If not quite an Orwellian night-mare, it was everything that a bad dream aspired to be. What was especially disconcerting was the oddness of working in organisations that had, seemingly independently of general moral norms, evolved regimens of multiple, complex rules, tailored to the survival of the organisation and its restrictive purposes.

Meanwhile, back in Ireland

It may be that the lower opinions of themselves, held by men-tal handicap nurses, contributed to the depressing attitudes they often displayed towards their charges. The deliberate forms of punishment were both sinister and disturbing, not only because systematic (and vicious), but also because of the contempt felt by those inflicting the punishments for what others might think. Carried out by a small number of male nurses under the tutelage of one of the monks whose religious order administered the hospital, these beatings were both an everyday occurrence and common knowledge to all who worked there. So as to maintain order amongst 30 or so severely handicapped boys, this monk, Brother Luke, had arrived at a point where he refused to rely upon medication as a sedative for unruly or aggressive behaviour (which at the time would have been routine) initiating, instead, a regime of unremitting slaps, punches and, on rarer occasions, sustained whippings with a thick leather belt (the latter item, normally, being a part of his religious garb). The transgressions that warranted this violence ranged from the trivial to the doubly trivial and so were legion. It must have been the sheer repetitiveness of the beatings that had dulled whatever capacity we might once have possessed to be shocked, amazed, or depressed. Yet we student nurses, although still bright-eyed and idealistic in other respects, seemingly adapted to it. We could not have become completely immune to it, I suppose, else I would hardly be writing this. Having said that, why did I not do something at the time?

Don't just stand there, do something

Why didn't any of us do something about it? I don't know. We were no different from other groups of 20-year-olds. On the whole idealistic, reasonably bright, religious up to a point, and wanting to 'do something for our fellow man' (which is why we were there in the first place). So that 'why we didn't do something' is the question that aches. I cannot recall any battle between the desire to take a moral stance as against the need to keep one's job. Nor do I recall agonised discussions among the students as to what we could say or do about it. Probably, we were helped by the sort of rationalising, which holds that knowing something is wrong is not quite the same thing as causing it to be wrong. Perhaps. The problem, however, and the thing that rankles most, is that nearly everybody, given sufficient pressure, yielded to the impulse to smack and slap even if, in most cases, this smacking was of the reactive, sometimes paternal/maternal kind and hardly in the same league as Brother Luke and his team. While the prevalence of this 'lesser' punishment was worrying enough on its own terms, it made any negative reactions to the brutality of Luke's regime all the more difficult. At the end of the day, people in glass houses shouldn't throw stones and that was the nub of the problem. For, although the majority of nurses behaved decently, the occasional smack seeming to spring from a genuine anxiety for a patient's welfare—akin to the instinctive smack that follows a child's attempt to run in front of a lorry—this (still unforgivable) 'lower level' of punishment made criticism of the harsher brutality virtually impossible. Although most would not have wanted it that way, a mixture of passive acquiescence (bordering on complicity) ensued, to some extent mitigated by apprehension of the likely consequences of objecting.

Students today

It is interesting to speculate about how students would react to such events today. Looking back on his life, the novelist Kingsley Amis was asked whether he might have done things differently. He replied that such questions are beside the point. To have acted differently, he said, would have meant being different. There is something to this, because it implies that if you do your best in the circumstances, then much more cannot reasonably be expected of you. Yet circumstances do matter and Amis's point doesn't quite account for why people, particularly in groups, can act out of character and behave immorally towards others, even grotesquely so. This raises the question of whether immoral behaviour comes about through individual choice, or from an interplay between individual choice and the coercive effects of social pressure. If we believe that today's students would publicly condemn violence against patients as unethical, this might be less to do with changes of character or temperament, but that dissidence is tolerated more than it was back then. Putting this another way, people today are less enamoured of traditional icons of power and authority; they possess a greater willingness to 'go public' if the source of their discontent ignores them, or reacts negatively to their criticism. In these respects, nursing practice has undoubtedly become better.

In the past, nurses were obsessed with subservience, suckers for an occupational socialisation in which a matron or charge nurse's word was law. On being posted to a new ward, we didn't ask about its nature or its patients, no: we asked who was in charge and what were they like. Where sufficient information could be gleaned about prospective sisters and charge nurses, preemptive measures could be worked out to deal with their foibles and quirks. This was a world of hierarchies, uniforms, rules, bath books, bowel books, nursing orders, and myriad punishments for anyone failing to live up to them. It was a symbiotic relationship in which a demoralised staff, lacking self-esteem, found solace in the restrictive regulations of their hospitals and its bosses. The temptation to be obedient and loyal was strong, and in many ways this was an easy option since it incurred a curious self-satisfaction in knowing that one belonged. Having said that, in coercive systems, matters are never so simple as having to obey rules. Some people find rules appealing, some people derive satisfaction from the safety and predictability they provide: well-oiled, authoritarian, organisations rob one of the need to think.

Outside information

Empirical investigations into conformity and compliance support these conclusions. Such investigations properly began when Solomon Asch (1952) showed how group norms exert a compliant effect on individuals who differ with their group on an item of perception. A typical experiment would involve persuading a group of students to indicate that one of a series of lines (drawn on paper) was longer when it, patently, was not. Any student, not 'in on the act', came under intense pressure to comply with the majority's perception. Subsequent studies showed that cultural factors played a significant role in these processes. For example, Perrin and Spencer (1981) demonstrated differences in compliance between university students and young offenders for similar tasks. The students were not as compliant as the offenders, particularly when the latter were tested in groups that included probation officers. It seems that the rate of conformity increases as a function of the socio-economic backgrounds of people, which influence the expectations they bring to bear on questions of conformity.

According to Festinger (1957), where a situation is novel, ambiguous, or vaguely threatening, social reality tends to be defined by the ideas and behaviours of others: it is the behaviour of others that 'clues us in' to the norms of a setting, the way it works. Festinger's ideas help us understand the situation of immigrant student nurses trying to contend with autocratic hospital regimes. Absolutely no measures were taken to acclimatise immigrant nurses into British culture or norms: they were just expected to get on with the job. The same, of course, holds true for students from the indigenous population, although to a lesser extent. The point is, when the social 'realities' of situations are constructed by others, it will take considerable self-assurance to challenge them: therein lies the strength of institutional practice. In extreme situations, such as the violent domain of Brother Luke, the pressure to comply would be even more difficult to resist.

Any old excuse

Yet we can see, I think, that while social conformity theories can work as retrospective 'explanations' of why people acted in a certain way, they can also sound like making excuses. Remember that, in the Asch experiments, most subjects knew perfectly well that their perception, as opposed to the group's, was 'correct', but complied so as to avoid inter-group conflict. Was there never a point in which they could have remained true to their own selves? However, a truer conformity can also occur where the subject comes to believe in and identify with the norms of the dominant group. Most of us operate in groups of varying size and with different degrees of cohesion and fidelity. From our families to our occupations, and all the way to the State, we develop allegiances that we try to differentially satisfy, both to our own and their satisfaction. Complexes of personality and circumstances combine with history and culture to provide human landscapes from which spring astonishing examples of human goodness, as well as evil. Obviously, it is the latter that now interests us, the juncture where individual responsibility merges with corporate need, or demand.

It has become commonplace to ask how Germany could have given rise to and sustained the Hitler machine. How could a cultured nation spawn concentration camps where millions were tortured and killed? How could Third Reich doctors and nurses conduct human experiments in the name of science—apparently operating under 'codes of conduct'—while still retaining some semblance of self-respect? Perhaps it was straightforwardly something to do with being German, at least at that time and under those conditions? This is still a common view and was the basis of a controversial essay on Germany by Sunday Times columnist A A Gill (1999). For Gill, the problem is not the war, which is forgivable enough, the unforgivable is the Final Solution, a crime that 'stands beyond credulity or forgiveness' (p23). For Gill, the tragedy is compounded by what he sees as the Germans 'running to the future', which is really a means of avoiding the past.

Alison O'Donnell (Mathiesen, 2000) is researching nurses' activities within the Nazi camps. Little work has been done on the role of nurses—most studies have concentrated on doctors—and the question that has preoccupied O'Donnell is how nurses could have participated in the mass euthanasia of mentally ill and handicapped people. O'Donnell believes explanations lie in their socialisation into Nazi beliefs over a period of time, so these nurses came to believe that their victims were unworthy of human respect, whereas the State had to be obeyed. That is, those involved off-loaded responsibility on to the State where, in the case of the Third Reich, the distinction between individual and regime became blurred. The scale of the brutality is well known to us: what jars, intuitively, is that nurses were intimately involved in the administration of Nazi medicine. Recently, some viewers expressed dismay when a television documentary contained interview footage with German ex-servicemen, who expressed no remorse for what they had done. One old man spoke of the exultation he still feels recalling the moment when the Fuhrer momentarily looked at him. This provoked some viewers to ask if these people had learned nothing. How could they so massively lack insight into what they had done? A possible answer, as theatre director and neurologist, Jonathan Miller, pointed out, is to recognise that they believed in what they did: why should they feel remorse for doing what they believed was right? If, in 'good' conscience, one does what is right, then how, at the same time, can one judge one's actions to be wrong? Imagine a solitary German soldier taking part in a massed Nuremberg rally. Imagine he becomes caught up in the frenzy of the crowd, losing himself to the mesmerising dictator with his rallying cries for war and destruction? Imagine that the soldier loses himself to the crowd, the whole of which is greater than the sum of its parts: can he then say that responsibility for his actions is not his alone? Can he say that he did the right thing in the name of the Fatherland? Before looking at this more closely we need to reprise an earlier and more fundamental question.

The Greeks

The question of whether one can knowingly do wrong was famously addressed by Plato, whose contention that 'no one does wrong willingly' is difficult to comprehend as, indeed, it was when Plato said it. What it means is that if I do something wrong, I do so because I did not know the right thing to do: I acted in ignorance. Part of the difficulty in understanding this is to realize that Plato was less interested in what constituted a good act, as much as in what constituted the good life: more accurately, perhaps, the 'good state to be in'. In other words, Plato envisages the moral agent as always striving to think his way through to the best decision possible. If one thinks something through long enough then a good, reasoned decision would result: the man of reason comes to know what is right; evil stems from ignorance. In modern philosophy, this question was taken up by Richard Hare. Hare (1963) believed that true fanatics are few on the ground, but that their power is manifold on account of their ability to whip up support from those who would not otherwise be fanatics themselves. By processes of propaganda, they mislead and inflame others into thinking and behaving in sometimes morally reprehensible ways.

People are misled because they fail to disentangle truth from falsehood: they become unable to 'distinguish genuine facts from those facts that are really concealed evaluations' (Hare, p185).

Hare contrasted this with the ideals of liberal Englishmen or Americans who are prepared to subject their ideas to argument and debate. In the case of the Nazis, Hare states that war was inevitable given their unwillingness to subject their views to argument. However, he then proceeds to ask what would have emerged had such a debate occurred. He surmised that liberal argument would have failed because what the Nazis did was 'extend an aesthetic style of evaluation into a field where the bulk of mankind think that such evaluations should be subordinated to the interests of other people' (p161). In other words, they put ideals before people. However, putting people before ideas seems to suggest that what is right is what benefits people and that might not, actually, be true. After all, we are prepared to kill Germans for our principles or, more correctly, in defence of them. Whether, like the Nazis, we would seek to exterminate people in pursuit of an idea is, perhaps, what separates us from them: the moral affront, says Hare, is not so much their ideas, as their putting them into practice.

Hare's discussion heralds the troublesome question of whether the Nazis knowingly did wrong, for, if they were capable of (monstrously) moving some human groups beyond that which morality ordinarily deals with, it would seem that they did not. Brecher (1998) critically discusses Hare's position in 'Getting What You Want?' (pp54–9). Specifically he returns to the Platonic notion of not knowingly doing wrong. He notes Lang's (1990) point that, because the Nazis attempted to conceal what they did, this must mean they were aware of their wrongdoing. However, says Brecher, that they knew that others would be affronted is not an acknowledgment of culpability. Cover-ups are about avoiding retribution. Similarly, in the case of Brother Luke, a moral cordon surrounded what went on, but this was in respect of being wary that 'outsiders' might pay a visit and cause trouble. Equally, the common phenomenon of the concentration camp guards inhabiting one moral world when at home, and another when 'at work', hardly suggests moral conflict if they had a regard for the people who inhabited these different places as valuable human beings. Lang contradicts this, stating that, of course, the Nazis knew that they inhabited the same moral world as everyone else and this means that they chose to do evil. Choice, by definition, involves rationality: questions of responsibility rest on the role that reason plays in motivating us to act. In the case of hospital brutality, there is evidence (DHSS, 1972; 1974) that people knew that bad things were happening, but were motivated by fear of retribution if they spoke out. The philosophical literature tends to emphasise the place of reasoning in these matters. In general, it neglects that psychological evidence that suggests—certainly in the case of institutions—that reason might not be the dominant factor in motivating us to act.

Festinger

Festinger's (1957) approach to this question was to account for discrepancies between thinking and behaviour. He called his theory 'cognitive dissonance'. Briefly, the theory holds that people prefer their cognitions, including those about their own behaviour, to be consistent with one another. When their cognitions are dissonant, people become uneasy and so strive to bring them back into uniformity. In an early investigation, Festinger and Carlsmith (1959) had subjects perform a very dull task and then persuade others that the task was actually 'fun'. Some were paid one dollar to do this, while others were paid 20 dollars. Surprisingly, those getting the one dollar revealed a higher approval of the dull task than those given 20. It seems that, in the absence of external justifications (in this instance the 20 dollars), or rather when there appears to be little justification for an unpalatable action, we change our attitude towards it. By making the object of our attentions less unpalatable, we bring our behaviour into line with our cognitions.

Whether Festinger's theory would account for behaviour under abnormal or extreme conditions is another matter. It seems as if people can be induced to support extreme brutality or oppression with relative ease, and we are not restricted to the Nazi example to make the point. I recall a phrase from my school history book about a group of British soldiers called 'Black and Tans', a name given to them because of the contrasting colours of their uniforms. My history book did not go into details, providing only the cryptic statement: 'These men were guilty of many lawless deeds'. I later discovered that, setting aside the exaggerations that grew about them over time, these lawless deeds included some killings of supposed Irish insurrectionists (see Kee, 1980). Again one asks: why? These were British soldiers, not German Nazis. Of course their actions bear little comparison to Nazi atrocities. However, the point is, that under certain conditions, an absence of moral controls, perhaps, or more precisely, a set of controls that permit extreme behaviour, most of us—at any rate most men—are capable of forgetting their 'better selves' and behaving badly. As we shall see when we turn to Milgram's work, Hare's 'liberal American and Englishman' seems more a product of academic discourse than anything else.

What Festinger does is provide a psychological mechanism that mediates the boundary between behaviour and thought. Where the problems of reconciling brutal actions becomes too much, we change gear attitudinally and make the object of our violence less worthy of consideration. So, when the nursing student found himself in new and vaguely threatening situations, the coercive effect would be to inculcate in himself the belief that whatever the violence done to patients, it did not merit the concern that would normally attend such brutality.

However, while at first sight plausible, Festinger's theory still seems insufficient to account for cases of extreme aggression or outright violence. It seems a paltry exercise when aligned with the great human tragedies of history. Historically, we have tried to define evil (such as the Nazis) as an 'enormity', a profoundly disturbing event that transcends psychology and even philosophy in its hideousness. There is much to this. However, in a series of experiments that an ethics committee would, nowadays, prohibit, Stanley Milgram

(1974) showed that, under certain circumstances, the average 'man in the street', and an American street at that, could inflict serious violence on others and all because asked to do so by figures of authority.

Milgram's experiments

Milgram persuaded subjects to administer electric shocks to people of such severity that some of the recipients—who were actors—screamed as if in great pain. Influenced by Asch's conformity experiments, Milgram wanted these to be less synthetic and more socially plausible. This was a sensitive issue: World War II had only just ended and memories of the Nazi atrocities were still very much alive. Before he began, Milgram had inquired of psychiatrists how many people would deliver the shocks, and they responded that only a small fringe of psychopathic types would do it. Confident himself that the compliant rates would be low, he toyed with the idea—quickly abandoned—of taking cross-measures between German and American subjects, no doubt hypothesising significant differences between them. In fact, many of his American subjects obeyed his instructions with relative ease, even in one celebrated instance when he informed a subject that the person on the receiving end had a bad heart.

One interesting finding was that subject's willingness to administer the shocks diminished as a function of closer proximity to their 'victims'. This proximity feature is important because, in Brother Luke's case, both the perpetrators and victims were in constant close proximity to each other. This is a puzzle: why should physical proximity inhibit cruelty within experimental settings while enhancing it in real life? Why didn't the abysmal fear on the faces of handicapped men stay the hand of people purporting to be nurses? It suggests that some differences may attend the artificiality of settings where violence occurs. The experimental setting allows the subject to feel, maybe, that some greater, perhaps wiser, mentality underpins what is going on, i.e. that it is in the name of science. What Millgram seems to have done is dangerously blur the lines between experiment and actuality such that, for some subjects, there came a point in which the balance tipped towards reality and they began to demur. Reality in this sense being the re-emergence of the everyday rules of moral engagements. Wardhaugh and Wilding (1998) suggest that the corruption of care occurs when normal moral concerns are set aside: they refer to Zygmunt Bauman's (1989) work to extend this point. Bauman had dealt with the question of proximity (of torturer and victim) by stating that the torturer puts the victim beyond the bounds of moral obligation. In Bauman's view, Jews 'ceased to be those others to whom moral responsibility normally extends' (p189). Exclusion leads to dehumanization, to what Wardhaugh and Wilding call 'moral invisibility' and this agrees with O'Donnell's view of how the Nazi nurses were able to do what they did.

Instrumental and hostile

Frude (1980) distinguishes between instrumental and hostile violence, the former being violence in the service of some goal, the latter the desire to inflict damage for its own sake. Milgram's subjects were instrumental in serving the needs of an experiment. So long as the experiment remained within certain artificial boundaries, they were able to proceed. On being exposed (by proximity) to those whom they were 'torturing' they refused in increasing numbers.

Luke and his assistants, alternatively, were in close proximity to their patients anyway. This is their habitat; they are already party to a setting where violence is the norm. Their violence is both instrumental and hostile; it serves the organisation, represented by Luke, but is also hostile inasmuch as genuine rage could attend their beatings, especially if the behaviour that had induced the beating was seen as a result of the nurses' failure to keep order.

The good brother

Brother Luke probably experienced no remorse when leathering handicapped boys, because he believed what he was doing was right, was in their interests. One can but speculate about what he conceived their 'interests' to be. It had to have something to do with 'good' behaviour: not good in any moral sense, because even he must have realised that these boys were incapable of sound moral reasoning. Rather, it had to be something to do with social etiquette, his desire to bring them to a standard commensurate with the **appearance** of good behaviour, maybe. To this end, he and his assistants would beat imperfections out of them and so force them into a semblance of good citizenship. I am not suggesting that this was an explicit formulation on their part, but that, in practice, this is what they appeared to be doing. From a religious perspective, these handicapped boys may have signified a failure on God's part; they were an affront, since they embodied a human frailty that was threatening, because inexplicable, to someone who believed that the perfection and perfectibility of God should be without limits. Whereas some would see in these handicapped people the faces of angels—their passage to heaven being ultimately guaranteed was a remark one often heard—in Luke's domain, they were an imperfection; an imperfection that could yet be redeemed at the hands of his hard and unremitting tutelage.

Luke's assistants belonged to a category of nurses called 'assistant nurses', and they performed at roughly the same level as Enrolled Nurses in Britain. For instance, they administered oral and intra-muscular medication although clearly not properly trained to do so. One of them, whether through world-weariness or sheer ignorance, had perfected a system whereby he dispensed quite complicated prescriptions by memorising the various colours and shapes of the drugs involved. So, for instance, patient B would get two small reds, two white ovals, one small purple and so on: he was helped in his task by the high proportion of anti-epileptic drugs which, when effective, are rarely altered.

There were about four of these assistant nurses and they operated at different degrees of brutality, but with the two males especially keen to punish. Something which they had in common with the rest of the hospital's nurses was a strong belief in what Heider (1958) calls 'dispositional attribution', the tendency to attribute motives to people's dispositions, while correspondingly playing down the part that circumstances play in human behaviour. Luke's assistants seemed especially prone to read capricious intent into even the most cumbersome blunders and emotional outbursts of their patients. On Saturday afternoons, the able-bodied patients congregated for a film show, always a welcome occasion for both staff and patients to relax and mingle. Luke's assistants, however, rarely relaxed: instead, they maintained a constant vigilance, relentlessly calling attention to this or that patient who might be about to misbehave in some way. Their method of dissuasion was hard (open-palm) slaps delivered to the back and temple regions of the head: variations on this were a single blow to the head or chest, their bunches of keys becoming effective knuckle-dusters.

The social audience

It also matters that these attacks were perpetrated in full view of whoever happened to be present, although some apprehension might attend the uninvited arrival of the Father Superior who was not a hitter. In general, however, Luke and his team remained virtually a law unto themselves, unencumbered by the attentions of others: indeed, their unconcern was well founded. In any event, a range of factors acted to form a fairly impenetrable boundary around their practices. For example, students were rarely allocated to Luke's ward and Matron, when on her rounds, studiously avoided entering it. It is easy to see all this as an example of 'see no evil, hear no evil', but, looking back, her reserve must have been intended as a negative comment of sorts, which is more than could be said about the rest of us. On the other hand, she was the Matron at a time when that role still counted for something: she should have acted more vigorously.

Frank's excuse

Frank Singleton was a charge nurse who had once worked for Luke and his rationale for taking part in some of Luke's sustained beatings is interesting. Throughout the hospital, 'bad behaviour' was common because many of the patients were epileptic. In the event that they had an epileptic seizure, all was well and good. Sometimes though, the seizure lay 'dormant' with the neurological disturbance taking the form of disruptive, 'epileptic equivalent' behaviour, which could last for hours. Persistent behaviour, such as this, warranted more than the usual reactive slaps with Luke insisting that the offender be held, spread-eagled, on the floor so that lashes could be delivered to the bare buttocks.

Frank's excuse for assisting in this took the form: 'I used to hold them down while he gave them the belt, but then I'd let them go saying "OK Brother Luke" as if to say 'that's enough' and at that he'd usually stop'. To Frank's way of thinking, I suppose, he was saving them from further punishment: in effect, a utilitarian argument that less pain is better than more. That he had aided and abetted the punishments seemed, to him, less of a crime since, by doing so, he had shortened the patient's distress. We each of us find our own way out.

Whistleblower extraordinaire

Of course, I made my protest, I became a whistleblower, of a type. During a visit by a psychiatric delegation from England, I took one of them aside and made vague allusions to 'things not being right', murmuring about a 'need to look beneath the surface', or words to that effect. Naturally, I did not give my name. My listener was 'all ears' even if I never heard from him again. But I was pleased with myself; I had spoken out; I was not like the others; my conscience was clear!

How feeble it all seems now; two minutes of conspiratorial chat to an Englishman who may well have thought I was deranged. Imagine! I was making allegations against a religious order renowned for its work with handicapped people,

that they were standing by while one of their number system-
atically brutalised patients.

Relief

It was with relief that I stepped aboard the Dublin ferry for
England, in the expectation that such things could hardly happen there. I was to be disabused of that notion. While there
was no equivalent of Brother Luke, an air of punitiveness surrounded much of the mental care of (especially) male patients.
What was different to Ireland was the growing public intolerance of such behaviour. From Ely Hospital to Whittingham,
from St. Augustine's to Farleigh and South Ockendon, inquiries into allegations of neglect proliferated; their revelations of
violence not just reflecting poor hospital conditions, but also
revealing a gratuitous violence. In the long run, these reports
hastened the end of the mental hospitals, which, for all their
supposed advantages (Jones 1972), had become little more
than medieval lockups where people could be abused in the
knowledge that they would stay silent about it.

You will not find these inquiries on the reading lists of
nursing courses. They hardly square with the triumphalist
assertions of today's professionals. Yet we do well to remain
cautious. Stanley *et al* (1999) note that almost 12 000 people
with learning disabilities remain in long-stay hospitals and, of
course, the number of those in alternative institutional care is
even larger. They quote Ramcharan (1998) that the potential
for abuse in these places remains real, especially for those with
the severest difficulties.

It was with both despair and dismay that I came across a
report in the Nursing Times (1999b) of two nurses struck off the
Nursing Register having been found guilty of beating learning
difficulties patients, having tied them to lavatories and generally humiliated them. I had thought that it was over, that the
violence had become a thing of the past. However, these cases
are not rare, as the accounts by Stanley *et al* (1999) show. Verbal
'assaults' of varying nuance and severity, as well as serious
neglect, are certainly common in the care of the elderly
(Coombes, 2001), as are 'techniques', such as unnecessary force

when sitting old patients down or lifting them up. Simply moving older people, as you would a chess piece, when its time for their dinner or bedtime, is also a typical manoeuver. In addition, nursing violence is also currently formalised by practices, such as 'control and restraint', the excessive use of drugs, and seclusion, to which we may now add the imminent threat of compulsory treatment in the community. These practices often proceed with little discussion or debate. In a series of interviews with the nursing staff of a forensic psychiatric unit (Clarke 1996), none of its 40 nurses expressed any irony or doubt at the presence of riot equipment for (potential) use in controlling patients. In general, the impetus to induce conformist behaviour is still strong: in terms of how it is organised and distilled (in law), it could even be said to be stronger.

A law to oneself

It is difficult for outsiders to appreciate the manner and speed by which enclosed communities became laws unto themselves, the peculiar ways by which a hermitage morality redefined patients as less worthy of the basic decencies and benefits of life. One would think that being in 'the high street' in the way that so many sub-units of the old asylums now are, would dissipate the bad old ways. However, it is the manner by which these units retain an asylum ideology that matters. The fact is too many of them still retain elements that characterised those asylums. The issue is about being judged. Institutions generate rules and these often lie in the direction of conservatism and restriction where patient's behaviours are concerned. However hard one tries, it is often difficult to escape the self-doubt that accompanies enlightened care against a background of implied censure from more organisationally 'aware' colleagues. No matter how hard one tries, the pressure to conform to what suits the institution is perpetually present. This is especially the case where existing conformity is high. Oppressive regimes become suspicious of even the slightest dissidence; it can open a can of worms.

What is to be done? Well, we need to attend to both social and innate factors. The greatest preventative measure against a punitive institutional culture is enhanced contact with the outside world. All communities should be denied the get out clause of being 'in the community'; they should be the community. Also, nurses' education might benefit more from a wider consideration of the social history of nursing than from its current preoccupation with humanistic counselling and 'the individual'. If, as the actor Joss Ackland recently said, we could unlearn the post-Thatcherite lesson of caring more for ourselves and less for others, then we might appreciate more what it must be like for people trying to live together in small, but still extant psychiatric institutions: we might, at least, give decency and reasonableness a chance. It may be that wrong-doers are ignorant of their own evil—which is a disturbing thought—but this does not lessen the evil one iota. In the case of the Nazis, a war was fought to keep the German empire at bay, albeit disturbing accounts continue to surface in terms of who knew about these atrocities and when they knew, and who did or did not do something about it. O'Donnell (Mathiesen, 2000) believes that some of the concentration camp nurses had 'blackened' or shut out from their consciousness what they were doing or had done. Others, she says, may have acted through fear of what would happen to them, if they did not comply. 'Nurses today', she says, 'need to beware of the slippery slope to complicity: they need to be guardians of their patients'. Of course, the scale of these outrages varies widely: however, the propensity to act detrimentally towards vulnerable groups is energised when everyday moral restrictions are removed, or overthrown by institutions that substitute, instead, their own concerns or ambitions.

Epilogue: the man himself

Brother Luke was short (surprise, surprise) and solid, not a superfluous bit to him. His shaved head (unusual then) suggested a pugilist perhaps; it certainly gave him a 'no nonsense' look that could be slightly intimidating. A daily swimmer, outdoors, winter and summer, he was not faint-hearted. A stickler for timekeeping and hygiene, he imposed these ideas on those over whom he had power. He seemed intelligent in a

7
A vocational exercise

*I*n a recent debate about nursing as a vocation (Nursing Times, 1999c), a nurse insisted that his vocational 'calling' meant that he 'gave his heart and hands, as well as his skills, to his patients'. Surprisingly, he said that he worked 'not for the hospital that employed him, but for himself' by which, doubtless, he meant self (regard), not self-aggrandisement. At one point he stated: 'nurses never have to ask themselves why their job is important, they know they are real people doing real jobs, they know what a vocation is'. No hang-ups about evidence-based practice here! This is a knowledge base that comes from 'within', from the self-assuredness of the individual practitioner. Such beliefs also afford the bearer an air of self-righteousness in their dealings with others and, thus, disavow any need for external validations of conduct. Interestingly, and perhaps not wishing to ditch 'reality' completely, this same advocate of vocation also thought that nurses should be adequately recompensed for their work.

His 'opponent' in the debate, a nurse-lecturer, described nursing as just a job, something that you become interested in, study for, get paid for and, ultimately, leave. Those claiming a vocation, he said, were merely satiating 'personal needs' and that bringing such needs into one's work could even interfere with patient care. Vocations are also bad, he insisted, because they weaken the claims of pay lobbies, diverting nurses from monetary and other occupational concerns. In addition, vocational nurses see their role as delivering 'basic care' and, while this commitment constitutes the heart of nursing, it leaves one open to undue influence from other quarters, namely medicine. Another criticism of vocation is that it operates as its own yardstick, apparently oblivious to external rules or standards for practice, whereas professionalism is about autonomous practice backed up by agreed standards or evidence.

Old ideas

The roots of this dichotomy are ancient. For Aristotle, the worthwhileness of a life depends on action, since it is little use having abilities if one chooses not to discharge them. The good person is a 'do-gooder': he is not paid to do good; neither is he good because of any praise he might win. Rather, he is, like Aristotle himself, a kind of unpaid savant or, better still, in Peter Mullen's (1983) phrase, someone whose virtue stems from 'virtuosity'. Aristotle's dictums, however, have the feel of being a 'tall order', probably because coming from a society where elitism was the norm. The modern parallel—not far off the mark—would be of a minority of nurses waxing lyrically about theoretical issues, while the majority of their colleagues constantly adapt to the increasing demands and complexities of practice. Practising nurses, on the whole, would seek to engage with the social, organisational, and technical require-ments that normally prevail in the workplace. Chief among these is the pre-eminent position of medicine and the scientific foundations from which it derives its power and authority. The nursing quest for a knowledge base—or evidence base as it is now fashionably called—takes place within this unenvi-able context.

Of course, there is no reason why goodness and good pay should contradict. Neither should a vocational disposition deflect nurses from professionally acquainting themselves with modern approaches to care. That said, vocational nurses do tend to play down personal recompense, emphasising instead the kinds of satisfaction that come from knowing one is living one's life according to good moral principles. On its own, however, goodness seems hardly enough to satisfy nurses who wish to be seen as practising from an evidence base: indeed, it seems difficult to conceptualise vocation as having any kind of evidence base at all.

Evidence base

It has become a truism, in some circles, that nurses should pro-vide evidence for the efficacy of their interventions. According to Brechin and Sidell (2000), evidence, in this context, usually means the sort derived from scientific studies: quantitative, analytic, and replicable.

A minority, however, have asked what should count as evidence: whether, in addition to empirically derived facts, other kinds of material might also count as evidence. To try to answer this, we need to examine the relationship between empiricism, science, and medicine. Empirical research seeks to discover the natural world, its laws and movements, through observation and testing. It assumes that an objective world exists independent of what knowledge we might have of it, and the business of science (and its methods) is to discover that world and measure it accurately. That which cannot be measured, such as human experience or value systems, lies outside this world. Notwithstanding major challenges to the philosophical assumptions of science, for instance, Popper's (1959) point that science doesn't establish truth, but falsifies it, or Kuhn's (1970) ideas about paradigm shifts, few deny that science provides the best tools by which to test beliefs about the physical world. If nurses are to account for their practice in evidence-based terms, then their research will need to be compatible with the scientific assumptions underlying evidence claims. Such a view, however, is inclined to overlook the fact that not all nurses admire this view of science and its evidence. As Bracken and Thomas (2001) point out, proponents of evidence-based practice fail to appreciate the different value systems that exist within nursing groups. Among psychiatric nurses, for example, a significant (albeit heterogeneous) group remains committed to using narrative forms within patient care. Important issues of control and ownership—of knowledge and resources—are at stake here. Utilising the narratives of self-advocating user groups, for example, could upset the control exercised by professional groups, if the latter were obliged to take these narratives as an additional evidence base. Interestingly, the Standing Group on Consumers in NHS Research (set up in 1996), which might have acted as a counter-balance to evidence-based studies, has omitted psychiatric patients, although, historically, this group has been as vociferous as any about health care issues. Some nurses have tried to harness the views of these patients as an alternative to facts-based empirical fare. Preferring to expand their relationships with patients into meaningful, although less easy to define, areas, they have created research strategies where the subjective world of patients becomes indispensable. Summarising these strategies, Professor Phil Barker (2001) states: 'Promoting the voice of the person in care is part of a paradigm shift in acute care: what appears to be a new mindset, however, is probably no more than the re-emergence of a much older attitude to nursing, one that has been starved of oxygen over the last ten years' (p39). Admiration for traditional values, however, invites criticism of 'living in the past' and, while there is nothing essentially wrong with that, it carries the implication of Luddite antagonism towards new ideas. The issue, though, is about the appropriateness of ideas and the manner by which they amplify as opposed to merely extend the nursing role.

Extended or expanded

The distinction between an expanded, as opposed to an extended, role for nurses is clear-cut. Extending the nurses' role is about the progressive acquisition of tasks previously carried out by others, for example, nurse prescribing. Among others, Gray and Gournay (2000) support a prescriptive role for psychiatric nurses in respect of psychotropic drugs; so, too, does Lipley (2000) for physical disorders, such as asthma and diabetes. Untangling the forces that drive nurses to extend their medical obligations is difficult. At a personal level, sheer ambition must play a part, either in terms of better rewards, professional satisfaction, or both. At a more general level, the economics of health care, especially its explosive costs, fuel the practice of re-allocating as many medical tasks as is feasible to lesser paid ranks who, in turn, will receive a better remuneration than **their** rank and file. Hence, for example, the emergence of consultant nurses with their higher than usual nursing, but still lower than usual medical, salaries. In respect of economics, it seems that as people's health needs expand

and the costs of doctor-focussed treatments increases, then pressure to extend the nursing role become irresistible.

The creation of NHS Direct (1997), a telephone service manned by nurses, is a prime example of these changes. This service is now a 'first port of call' for many sick people. It places nurses at the front line of diagnosing patient's problems and suggesting possible remedies for what ails them. It is disliked by many medical practitioners, but, because it has yet to be fully assessed, it is difficult to evaluate its present functioning: the Secretary of State for Health, Alan Milburn, likes it a lot. For those nurses committed to nurse prescribing, the question of whether NHS Direct is about medical economics and the transformation of nurses into quasi-medical practitioners will be ignored, as nurses continue to emulate their more powerful medical colleagues. It is my contention that the assumption of a prescribing role, administering injections, drips or thermometers, or diagnosing patient's illnesses is, basically, an appropriation of medical obligations and practices.

Expanding the **nursing** role, however, is a different matter. In order to speak meaningfully of an expanded role, nurses need a knowledge base that differentiates them from medicine and other disciplines. In other words, an expanded role is about showing how nursing differs from what other disciplines do. Whether such differences would be expressed in terms of a knowledge or skills base, or whether nursing could describe itself in some other way (see Davies, 2000) is a vexed, perhaps insoluble, question.

Doctors and nurses

For now, I propose to look at the settings where nursing takes place, so as to further tease apart some of the boundaries between doctors and nurses. From observations of actual practice, Allen (1996) found little disagreement between these two groups. Yet, when she examined 'the nursing literature', she was struck by repetitive and contradictory declarations by nurses that they were, indeed, professionally separate from doctors. Both findings can hardly be true. In fact, Allen's findings are not surprising because, at practice level, little has fundamentally changed between doctors and nurses, although, as Hart (1999) points out, nurse writing slyly ignores the interdependence of medical/nursing care within hospital settings. This is not new: Desmond Cormack (1983: p11) noted almost 30 years ago that, 'the prescriptive role of the nurse (found in the literature) does not always match the limited descriptive accounts which exist'. The discrepancy occurs because academic nurses seek to prescribe a (phantom) nursing knowledge free of the 'restrictions' of medicine. Whereas, in hospitals, rank and file nurses utilise their watered-down medical expertise, as a means of sustaining their collaborative alliance with the medics. Their overriding concern is about doing a practically difficult job and doing it well. These nurses cater to individual patients and, while they accumulate expertise (from experience), they do not seek to generalise from it in any theoretical way. One suspects that when delivering 'basic nursing care', they will accept the assurances of patients that things are better or worse. In effect, these assurances qualify as an audit of efficient care, their 'evidence base'. Of course there are difficulties here, not the least of which is the discrepancy between patients feeling better and being better: these are not mutually exclusive but the relevance of each may affect professional groups disproportionately. Nursing is perhaps to do with making people feel better, more comfortable, relaxed, resigned, or determined. Medicine is about these things, too, but it also seeks causal explanations for the patient's discomfort, etc., and, whenever possible, ways of curing it. In some instances, this division may be too neat: some nurses, for example, working in areas such as incontinence or sexual health clinics, may assume an educational and supportive role that appears to fill a gap between what medicine can offer or what people could do for themselves. This post-diagnostic 'nursing' may be where some nurses might achieve autonomous practitioner status.

For the majority, however, the distinctions between vocational and professional nursing holds true. Clearly, if difference exists between nurses, then the nature of their evidence-bases will also differ. The vocational nurses, who nurture patients through pain or distress, may have difficulties accounting for their actions in evidence terms: what kind of evidence demonstrates the 'effectiveness' of caring for a dying person in the **'act' of dying**? Finding out what that might be would mean going beyond what normally passes as evidence.

Philosophical view

Roger Scruton (1995), who should know, says that philosophers take inquiry beyond evidence-based considerations and rightfully so. Although science tries to explain the causal factors that link events, questions may still be asked about the scientific process itself, questions, such as, what counts as science and what constitutes the evidence upon which it bases its inquiries. Nurses, therefore, are entitled to inquire about the nature of evidence, especially if they reckon that aspects of nursing are at odds with the kinds of evidence valued by scientists. As with the dying patient, however, the problem is knowing how to make qualitative or narrative-based information explicit, how to communicate it in ways that make sense to a range of interested parties.

Work with patients that refers to feelings and value systems can be difficult to systematise or test, just as communicating non-behaviourist and non-tabulated data can be a problem. The National Service Framework for Mental Health (Department of Health, 1999a) lists only those nursing interventions supported by empirically derived evidence, specifically cognitive behaviour therapy, dialectical behaviour therapy, and psycho-social interventions, all of which lay claim to objectivity, systematic description, and quantitative outcomes. Since only a minority of nurses are trained in these, the implication is that most nurses are operating outside of evidence-based practice: the underlying (moral) implication being that non evidenced-based practice is ineffective in terms of 'treatment' outcomes, as well as lacking in accountability to those who pay for it. Public accountability being the order of the day, interventions that lend themselves to numerical or behavioural measurement will win approval from purchasers of health care who, naturally enough, like to see what they are buying. Measuring the quality of care, however, may be problematic where nurse/patient relationships contain elements normally associated with human passion and moral belief. Nurses form attachments to their patients—think of the possibilities for this between, for example, children with learning difficulties and their carers. That being so, how would you tease apart the effects on a child's development of, let's say, behavioural techniques as against the emotional regard that both patient and nurse have for each other?

For Paley and Shapiro (2001), the central question is exactly what change is brought about by therapy, as opposed to the provision of warmth, trust, and respect? Taking note of Lambert's (1992) finding that only 12 to 15% of patients receiving a specific therapy—as opposed to a control group not receiving any—showed an enhanced positive outcome, they reasoned that good outcomes reflected as much the personality of the therapist as the specific therapy used. Such reports, however, gain little credibility in today's climate of factual, accountable research. As Repper (2000) points out, 'specific interventions, with proven effectiveness, have gained increasing value and are seen, by many, to be the essential tools of mental health nursing' (p577).

Virtue its own reward?

How, therefore, should society respond to a nursing practice that owes more to moral, social, and spiritual imperatives than it does to facts about the physical world? Consider someone who jumps into a river to save someone from drowning. Where the jumper cannot swim, heroic failure seems an admirable quality and there is something rather grand (and immeasurable) about such acts. The analogy is with someone who is dying and there is nothing further, of a curative nature, to do; nevertheless, nurses respond. There is an element within nursing that regards, as immoral, any unwillingness to help if helping would lead to an individual feeling better. Whereas, in the case of medicine, to implement an ineffective therapy would be immoral: medicine that does not 'work' is of no use.

Nursing, it seems, does not have to demonstrate the same kinds of therapeutic efficacy. Nor, on these grounds, must it corroborate its practice by facts-based evidence, especially when its practice addresses the experience and the implications of their patient's illness and not just the illness alone. Nurses do need knowledge of what ails their patients, but this knowledge is not (in a nursing context) an end in itself. Rather it is a way of helping people cope better with their illnesses. Approaches that look to vocation, therefore, may best describe what nursing is, because they move discussion beyond medicine in terms of how best to deal with the problems that illness brings.

Administrators, of course, will continue to demand efficiency and cost effectiveness from nurses. As such, they will legitimise nurse prescribing, favour randomised controlled trials, and continue to regard evidence-based data as the *sine qua non* of efficient practice. But is this inevitable? Surely it should be possible to inform medical administrators that nursing is also about caring for people in indeterminate and unaccountable ways. Tschudin (1999: p51) provides an example of a nurse discussing his relationship with his learning disability patient: 'I know I have made a difference in his life, but it is not something that can be measured. The difference lies in our friendship, based on equality and mutual respect. We give each other something special. I know it and he does, too.' This befriending of patients is not without its aims and objectives: it is about assisting people to live adequately in society: it is about establishing confidence and self-esteem, as well as a willingness to take risks with other people and organisations. It is also, for example, about ridding society of elements antagonistic to people with psychiatric problems, while substituting, wherever possible, what is most conducive to well-being. The impetus for such a programme could hardly be sustained by controlled trials alone, or the kinds of scientific thinking that reduces individuals to the 'level' of their pathology. Part of the nursing challenge is to articulate the kinds of work that supports the social and psychological well-being of patients. Perhaps recognising the political and economic factors, which underline such considerations, is to subscribe to a concept of vocation by another name. Whereas to forego the modernist sin of vocation is to limit—and I do mean limit—one's interventions to this or that therapeutic enterprise. One sees the contrast dramatically in the nursing care of dying patients, where the wisdom (for example, of a family member—or the patients themselves) recognises that someone's 'time has come' in opposition to well-meant, but fruitless medical effort. Thus, also, does the vocationally minded nurse transcend 'the physical' so as to help individuals who are either in pain or facing questions of life and death.

The nurse as therapist

In his book 'Nursing as Therapy' (1998), McMahon says that nursing is not only about making people feel well, but about making them well: nursing, he believes, is therapeutic and the caring function is now insufficient to account for what nurses do. Even when all medical aid is spent and nursing comes into its own—as reflected in the prescriptive phrase 'all nursing care'—McMahon asserts that this is not enough. Nursing, instead, must be 'a major force for achieving health for the patient' (p3). For McMahon, this discussion about vocation is an academic exercise, because 'nursing is what nursing does'. What nursing does is connect with evidence-based practice within an economic system that requires it to take on what were previously medical tasks, resulting in a nursing profession 'that leads to wellness, to beneficial outcomes for patients' (p5). McMahon acknowledges that, 'on the face of it, many of these new roles are substitutions of doctors with nurses and, therefore, not really nursing roles' (p16). The problem is, as Smith and Agard (2000) note, that 'despite considerable efforts, the nursing profession has been unable to claim a territory, which belongs to nursing alone' and that, as a result, 'the work that nurses do expands and contracts in response to external demands' (p211). This suggests that nursing is a formless occupation, unable to resist pressures that prey upon its lack of professional autonomy. The nursing weakness—if weakness it is—is a lack of clarity in respect of its occupational obligations. Conversely, this is precisely what vocation is; an indefinite commitment to human welfare, which is only partly determined by occupational factors.

What do nurses actually think?

Does the good nurse have a vocation? For that matter does the bad? For example, religious convictions might lead some nurses to decry certain actions. Roman Catholic nurses (among others) are provided with a conscientious objection clause that allows them to withdraw at the point of abortion. Other nurses might take part in abortions with few doubts as to the goodness of their actions. Such nurses are not acting immorally in contexts where abortion is acceptable. In any event, both pro- and anti-abortionist nurses act as they do because they care. The reason this is a conundrum is because, as Peter Allmark (1995) says, it is not enough to say that one cares, one must stipulate what it is one cares about; the object of caring is basic to its evaluation. As such, an 'ethics of caring' is profoundly mistaken because bad, as well as good actions, stem from the impetus to care. In cases where moral or emotional commitment is strong, it may be particularly salient to ask about the nature of the object of attention. If one's vocation is to minimise human misery, such a calling could support involvement in a range of activities, not all of them morally legitimate. That being so, it may help us to examine terms such as vocation, caring, and calling in the light of their capacity to obscure activities of doubtful worthiness. Arguably, a deeply held vocation could lead to self-righteousness; a commitment to 'standards' could as easily ride roughshod over people's needs as could a cruel or uncaring approach. Recently, the polemicist, Christopher Hitchens, criticised the standards of care provided by Mother Theresa and her religious order as inadequate, the inadequacy resulting, possibly, from the unworldliness of their religious calling. Whatever the validity of these criticisms, they suggest that declarations of vocation are not enough: one needs to examine the practical implications of vocations as they are routinely applied so as to be sure that the neglect of one (temporal) thing is not happening in the name of a (spiritual) other.

Difficulties

An initial difficulty with the idea of calling is, calling from whom? If the calling is from God, then where does this leave atheist nurses? Perhaps they have been called, but do not yet know it? Or they may believe that their 'calling' comes from socialist principles, their dedication a product of their desire to benefit people within a national health service. The latter could be construed as God 'working in mysterious ways', although they would hardly think so.

In a recent exchange between myself and Professor Jean Watson (2000), the Professor advocated a 'transpersonal approach' to nursing that leaned heavily on spirituality, stating that spirituality was endemic to the 'healing process'; that it was the 'essence' of nursing. My response was to restate a Marxist-Leninist position. 'Might not nurses motivated by a socio-political conscience be as good, as effective, in their practice as any other?' It is not as if there aren't non-religious moral theories that inform ethical action. Kantian ethics, for instance, provides a set of moral imperatives, which denote moral actions as valid providing one can wish that everyone in the same circumstances follow the same action. In effect, 'Do unto others', but with the religious dimension left out.

Actually, following this principle, if people were to give themselves selflessly to others—as vocation demands—then who would produce the wealth by which nations prosper? More specifically, what happens if vocation conflicts with the personal obligation to earn one's living? Does a calling mean that one gives of oneself to the point of self-exploitation, or the exploitation of others? Exploiting others might occur in cases where selfless devotion to one's job leads to the neglect of family and friends. Or, it might occur when selfless devotion to patients gives them expectations that cannot be met by others who are less committed. The point is that if a person believes they are called, then they will inevitably view 'good nursing' as also 'called', so that what they do becomes good by definition. If what they do requires self-sacrifice as, indeed, if they are called, it must, then they may assume that others can have such sacrifices demanded of them. Hence, the uncomfortableness of ordinary nurses when exposed to the 'high standards' of vocationally committed nurses.

The sacred

In her espousal of transpersonal nursing, Professor Watson draws attention to 'the sacred', an element of the relationship between nurse and patient that, if not religious, is redolent of mystery. The sense is of an invisible 'presence' residing within the nurse/patient relationship. Downe (1990) also points to 'immeasurable elements' in nursing, stating that these elements constitute its 'being'. Further, he says, the quality of caring cannot be analysed. Well, quite. The problem with this kind of theorising is that its unworldliness leads to an abandonment of real-world explanations and, while excessive attachment to factual data can be just as defeating, one can also go too far in an opposite direction. Extremes can often resemble each other and, often, little enough separates vocational dedication from the pursuit of professionalism. Both positions have the nurses' ambitions in common and not the welfare of patients. Downe, for instance, says that 'A higher status for ourselves will come of its own accord, if we are recognised for our caring and dedication, in other words for our vocation' (p24). This sounds fine except that the essence of vocation is supposed to be that it eschews gratification or reward? A life without reward seems psychologically implausible and, indeed, we have become used to nurses demanding pay increases and better conditions. The present image of nursing as a university-based (academic) activity is also relevant here. In the light of this, Redfern (2000) argues that concepts of nursing must change and 'it may even be appropriate to lose the title "nurse" in some circumstances. We have done well,' she says, 'to have held on to the activity called nursing for so long' (p21) A higher, quasi-medical, activity beckons. But if this is true, who will carry out what has, until now, constituted the basic tasks of nursing?

Did you call?

It appears that many nurses do not see their role in vocational terms. Mackay (1998), in a rare study, discovered that only eighteen percent of her respondents saw their work in these terms. She dubbed this minority the 'nursing come what may' group. Interestingly, a larger group (twenty-eight percent) saw nursing as 'just a job', equating job satisfaction with good pay and with frequent (wistful) allusions to 'the private sector'. Mackay's sample also contained a number of 'compound' views. For instance, some listed pay as important, but also named 'service to others'. Mackay also discovered a remarkable bias against academia whenever 'good nursing' was described, as well as repeated concerns about the 'character' of nurse recruits. Close analysis of Mackay's paper shows that, while the majority rejected the 'vocation' tag, time and again they described their work in ways that suggested 'calling' rather than professionalism. Phrases such as 'It's something worthwhile'. 'It's not just a job. It's what I always wanted to do' were repeated over and over. These statements, by Mackay's subjects, underpin Raatikainen's (1997) definition of vocation, which she uses interchangeably with calling. A calling, she says, is a determination to serve altruistically; it is a 'deep internal desire' to choose a profession, 'which a person experiences as valuable and considers her own' (p1111). The person 'hears a call' and responds altruistically, with fidelity, devotion, a commitment to 'being there' and so on. With a calling, says Raatikainen, nurses help people 'with their hands, their heads, but especially with their hearts'. Unsurprisingly, nurses who claimed such a calling rated their jobs as more worthwhile (than the non-vocation groups) and believed that they were better at giving 'basic nursing care'.

Anathema

Naturally, any talk of vocation is anathema to nursing professionalisers and, particularly, to the educationalists. According to Meerabeau (1998), nurse educationalists have spawned programmes markedly at odds with the realities of nursing practice. Others are more strident. Warren and Harris (1998) present a no-nonsense demand that nurses abandon their educational reforms, re-adopt their vocational role and return to bedside nursing. For Warren and Harris, the modern nurse wears Doc Marten boots, mouths a spurious language of 'care' and dreads the prospect of attending the bedside of sick patients. In other words, they have been 'educated' out of all responsibility for sick people:

'The very first aim of the nursing reformer, therefore, must be the return of the student nurse to the bedside, not as an observer, but as a member of staff, owing her loyalty to a hospital, a place where the sick are treated, not to a distant campus'.

(p32)

Although some nurses might happily agree, these criticisms are the hallmark of populist right-wing prejudices against 'female nurses who have gotten above themselves, drifted too far from 'service', become too concerned with issues of socio-professional status. This anti-women stance can sometimes seem comically out of touch:

'Twenty years ago student nurses could join a hospital to which they could offer what advertising men today call 'brand loyalty'. You were a St Thomas, a Great Ormond Street, or a Manchester Royal Infirmary trained nurse. Pay was awful, conditions were hard, but you were in a family, you were at 'your' hospital doing what you wanted to do, nursing the sick from the day you started.'

(p25)

Presumably the low pay didn't matter since, with any luck, you would marry a doctor and have children: or, you could eschew marriage altogether and become a ward sister, selflessly ministering to 'the sick' while crucifying the poor students who dared to take some time off because sick.

Falling off

So why is the concept 'vocation' not more widely used? Remarkably, even among ecclesiastics, its usage is declining. One reason for this is that sociological research tends to investigate professional issues and vocation simply does not fall within this material picture. Also, a romanticised view of nurses as purveyors of 'sweetness and light' diminishes the functional and medically-instrumental aspects of their roles. To remain a workable concept, therefore, vocation has to capture something of both worlds, the commitment of the individual as well as the collective, occupational responsibility to society at large. For many nurses, recent years have seen a shift away from personal commitment to collective concerns, although whether at the expense of professional obligations remains debatable.

Vocation has traditionally been about 'one's vocation in life', something that transcends one's job, an investment over and above the level of what is recompensed. If vocation is not its own reward, it is certainly not about obtaining reward whatever form reward takes. Such thinking is rarely far from the minds of governments and health administrators. In 1987, Trevor Clay charged that 'vocational nursing' was often used to justify low pay and poor conditions and, in a 1990 UK recruitment prospectus, nursing students were informed that their 'payment' would rest less on financial reward than on emotional satisfaction (Smith and Agard, 2000). The problem is to marry this up with Wallace's (1987) finding, later corroborated by Mackay (1998), that many nurses find the intrinsic nature of the work more important than salary or conditions.

Unsurprisingly, perhaps, most recruitment campaigns are directed at females who, according to Firby (1990), seem more likely to choose occupations that involve caring for people. Whether, as Benner (1984) would argue, nurses should utilise this caring paradigm in opposition to male power structures, with their exclusivity and specialities, is a moot point. It does seem awfully difficult to see how something as fluid as caring, something that does not require a specialist knowledge, could lead to the social recognition and economic recompense that many nurses seek. This is the paradox of vocation: to give one's services without putting a price on them invites the consideration that such services may not be worthwhile. Yet, this is not true for nursing whose intrinsic worth is generally admired. The problem is that this admiration rarely extends to decent pay awards or improved working conditions. On the one hand, nurses have no need of material reward because 'committed'; on the other, there are just too many of them. Far too many to warrant appropriate financial recompense, none so many as to merit approval bordering on reverence.

8
A question of language

There comes a point in respect of some things when anger inclines to weariness, and you have to ask if it really is worth the candle. I am referring, to endless nursing papers that proceed as if nursing was synonymous with general nursing, as if psychiatric nursing did not exist. Psychiatric nurses are not identical to general nurses; important elements separate them. It would be a mercy, therefore, if the latter would commence their articles, papers, books and discussions by stating which branch of the profession they are talking about. Psychiatric nurses, as a rule, do this: others should follow.

Such was my reaction to Professor June Clark's (1999a) account of the International Committee on Nursing Language and its work. Apparently, this committee's mandate was to evolve and standardise a language of nursing for world-wide use. It was not that Professor Clark's paper was poorly thought out or badly written, nor, even, that it failed to address questions of importance to nurses. Rather, its ambitions (in respect of universal language systems) seemed naively unrealistic, as well as being at odds with how language is currently used. My view was that Clark's paper would have taken a different turn had it included psychiatric nursing in its deliberations because, if any 'language system' has dominated modern nursing, it is surely the humanistic dialogues of Carl Rogers and Abraham Maslow. While some of this language—unconditional positive regard, non judgementalism, self-actualisation—has come to epitomise nursing, especially in its contemporary guise as a 'caring profession', it is psychiatric nursing that possesses greater legitimacy in its use. Currently, general nurses [more specifically an elitist group within this division] seem especially keen to adopt this language as part of its determination to define nursing separately from medicine. Professor Clark and her team appear to have missed this point.

In terms of nursing separating from medicine, the question of whether cultural settings 'control' language or vice versa becomes salient. From the vantage point of nursing, either explanation will suffice because what matters is that the remit of nurses is to address the needs of sick people in treatment settings. Despite attempts by nurse educationalists to promote community-based prevention, the dominant language of treatment settings continues to be medical in nature and this is not, in my view, debatable. The idea that, within medical/surgical settings, some kind of holistic philosophy would carry equal weight in a way that would impede medical necessity is slightly ridiculous. This is at the heart of the nursing problem: nursing cannot have a medical language since another profession already has that. Any nursing language that develops, as a medical alternative, requires to be different from medicine and this is fine if it does not seek to operate in medical settings. Of course, the broader concerns of contemporary nurses, for example care planning or ethical issues, enables a more comprehensive nursing care to proceed and the days of ritualist or ill thought-ought practice are over. However, the point about medical dominance (within treatment centres) remains valid.

The heart of nursing

The heart of nursing seems to be some kind of (tautological) disposition to care; at base level, nursing differs from other disciplines in its moral obligations to respond to human ills in the first instance. That is, in the absence of defined techniques or specified (anticipated) outcomes, nurses respond to human frailty anyway. Such responses, of course, may be knowledge-based inasmuch as they involve techniques. However, these techniques define other disciplines more than they do nursing. Within nursing, the impulse to respond stems more from value than epistemological systems. A problem with language occurs because of the difficulty in articulating nursing interventions without lapsing into medical terminology. The holistic/humanistic language that has come to characterise much recent nursing discourse, denotes nurse-patient relationships as central to care, and not the implementation of medical skills. Not surprisingly, some nurses seek comfort within the comparative certainties of the medical approach with its authoritative, technical language. Equally, others are adamant that these technical certainties spell disaster because they dehumanise the patient nurse experience.

Poorly understood

According to Professor Clark, nursing is poorly understood and so, therefore, undervalued. She says that, while these mis-understandings take different forms, essentially they boil down to the question, 'What is nursing'? Correctly stating that language does not allow precise descriptions of what nurses do, she further avers that, since 'we cannot name it, we cannot research it'. Well, I think that we can research it, albeit not with the quantitative precision sought by her International Language Classification Team. Even if appropriate, quantitative approaches fail to account for the relationship components of nursing. To measure relationships, some form of qualitative research is needed. The problem with qualitative studies is that, because their results are in narrative form, they possess nothing like the validity, control, and precision of quantitative approaches and, consequently, are seen by some as somehow second best, a kind of amateur research. However, such studies provide extremely valuable descriptions of the social settings of care and often suggest improvements or change. Whether nursing ultimately accepts qualitative research as a basis for its knowledge, or chooses quantitative (medicalised) systems instead, only time will tell. Certainly, if nursing is about relationships, then I cannot see how quantitative indices could explicate much that would be meaningful.

An instrument of care?

The aim of the International Language Classification Team is to produce just such a quantifiable language system and encode it within a computer programme. I am unsure here, if the classification team are confusing information with knowledge. The two are distinct. Computer systems are fountains of information, not fonts of knowledge, and it is the urgent need for a conceptual knowledge that preoccupies the thinking of general nurses. Also, in psychiatric nursing, where the issue is to establish human contact as a pre-requisite of growth and change, the introduction of computerised language systems seems faintly unbecoming. In defending the classification team's work, Professor Clark described other classification systems that had played variable, but significant roles in health care. Such systems, however, are invariably quasi-medical in nature, depending on pre-existing assumptions about the validity of cluster and syndrome approaches to knowledge formation. Moreover, if one examines the medical/psychiatric system most commonly used (the DSM IV), what is irksome about it is precisely its precision, the way that it excludes the experiential from human problems. So as to offset the criticism that this is what the reductionist language (of science) does, Clark suggested that it was not language that determined nurses' interactions with patients, but, instead, the care plans that many nurses now use to govern their interactions. Yet, she then stated—as she must—that such care plans are normally constructed from language. However, it is the nature of the language used that is the problem. An example of language misuse involves the stigmatising of mentally ill people. Without wishing to deny the reality of mental illness, psychiatric language can exert a determining influence on the lives of mentally ill people. True, compression of terms may be necessary; a professional dictionary of sorts is needed. Yet psychiatric nursing ennobles itself when it renders the experiences of ill people through the ordinariness of their language. The challenge is to understand their story. In psychiatry, as Tom Szasz says, we seek to encounter people, not decipher them through clinical concepts, information systems, or dispassionate language. There is a particular need to recognise the extent of the differences that exist between psychiatric and other medical-nursing spheres. In both cases, the restorative processes are going to be quite different. While there might be similarities, for example crash victims who face a lifetime being wheel-chair bound must attempt to overcome profound psychological difficulties, psychiatry becomes bound up with the very identity of patients as they attempt to define or re-define who they are. It is these considerations that render apart the relevance of language narratives in respect of the different branches of nursing. Psychiatric nurses have no choice, no way of avoiding the patient's story as the central determining event in his or her accounts of their history. When conventional psychiatry subjects that story to diagnosis and physical treatments, it often does so by utilising the language of compulsory care. Whereas, in general nursing, the preoccupation with language is either in the service of professionalisation—as in the International Language Classification Team endeavour—or as part of the determination to avoid medical dominance. Since this is an unrealistic exercise, and given that nursing is by and large a non-definable activity, general nurses have, on the whole, ended up floundering in a welter of idealistic posturing; the International Language Classification Team exemplifies that posturing.

Super-talk

I simply don't believe that an international language can take account of what nursing is in practical terms. Nursing people involves the formation of a relationship comprised of psycho-social complexes. The variability of nursing, wherein no two encounters are alike, is hardly fertile ground for what the International Classification Team are trying to do. I am baffled as to what the practical applications of such a classification would be. If, as June Clark says, the system is designed to communicate the meaning of nursing from an external, abstract, internationalist perspective (our very own nursing Esperanto), then this has little to do with nursing in practical terms.

In Professor Clark's view, my concerns about nursing language are different to those which concern the classification team. 'We are talking', she said, 'about different kinds of language used for different purposes'. Yet she also says: 'the purpose of this language and its documentation is to communicate with others who share the care of a particular patient to ensure coherence and continuity of care'. Well, which is it to be? Does the proposed international classification relate to actual care of patients, or is it some external super-system that comments upon and communicates a 'caring language'? If it is the latter, then how does it do it? Casey (2001), writing about a new European Language Association, says that a phrase, such as 'spinal procedure', is not much use in a medical record, if it is not specified as 'lumber puncture', and of course she is right. However, when she points to the potential mix-up between 'non-compliant' and 'chooses not to do', she ignores the moral imperatives that accompany these phrases, and the fact that 'non-compliant' could be the kind of diagnostic sleight of hand, which, in effect, denies patients their rights. That is to say, the patient is not seen as choosing for himself, but is deemed to 'have' non-compliance, this being indicative, somehow, of abnormality. If patient's choices accord with professional requests or directives, then 'compliance' is not an issue: unlike non-compliance, compliance does not exist in the psychiatric vocabulary. What matters is that the kinds of formal terminologies sought by Casey and the Association for Common European Nursing Diagnoses, Interventions and Outcomes would quash the kinds of political and moral subtleties that infuse psychiatric language.

Imposing concepts

Rather are these language classifications another example of that determination to impose taxonomies, of excessive elegance, on an occupation whose practising members are singularly uninterested in intellectualising away the practical nature of their origins and status. The taxonomy of caring has, by far, exercised the most influence in recent years. In effect, caring is elevated to the status of a philosophy (or science) by what, in my view, counts as some of the most circuitous and self-deluded writing of the century. Space permits only one or two examples of the genre. Take for instance Chinn and Kramer's (1999: p5) statement that 'personal knowing in nursing' is 'the inner experience of becoming a whole, aware, genuine self'. In a remarkably similar vein to humanistic psychology, they go on: 'One does not know about the self, one strives simply to know the self'.

There are two problems with this. To begin with, the validity of a concept, such as 'the self', is extremely problematic, something that is ignored by many nurse writers, as well as nurse education curricula. Second, there occurs a 'reality shift' whereby it becomes hard to see what the practical applications of 'the self' could be within surgical/medical settings.

This is not to deny that treatments should take place within a context of respect, kindness, and understanding. However, that we need much more than the ordinary decencies of life to ensure treatment occurs in a civilised way is questionable. Indeed, within many psychiatric settings, if we could deliver a nursing care roughly synonymous with providing patients with the ordinary civilities of life, we would be, at least, serving them well. This, of course, would require a shift away from theory and professionalism, as well as the acceptance of an advocacy role based on civil rights and the entitlement of patients to a good social existence. While, at first sight, this might resemble contemporary rhetoric about holistically motivated healthism [current nurse education emphasising community-based health and prevention programmes], it is, in fact, different. Approaches to nursing that are fuelled by holism are the hallmark of elitist groups, whose ambitions far outstrip those of the majority of nurses whose job it is to make clinical settings work. Mackay (1998), for instance, shows how the aspirations of general student nurses still lie in the direction of clinical settings and away from preoccupations with academia or intellectualising. As Meerabeau (1998) observes, 'the preparatory socialisation of nurses is currently discrepant with reality and students are disconcerted to find themselves in the lecture room or out "in the community" rather than on the ward' (p83). Given the practicalities of treatment settings, it ought to be possible to construct education programmes that take account of this.

For some, however, associating nurses with sick people in treatment settings smacks of a stereotype: it is an image that is anathema to the 'new nursing'. But whether the 'new nurses' like it or not, hospitals are here to stay. True, the nature of how we use them alters over time, and hospitals may well become, as they were before; more informal, more community oriented. True, midwifery comfortably operates without recourse to hospitals (provided the medical implications allow it) and mental hospitals have been virtually replaced in all but their acute, forensic and emergency forms. But it is romantic nonsense for general nurses to seek a world where the patient's pathology is side-tracked by some nebulous holistic enterprise.

Project 2000

Project 2000 was the supreme achievement of 'the new nursing' in Britain. Although some of its most cherished provisions are now being jettisoned (Munro, 1999), there remains a stolid avoidance of the real reasons behind this change back to more traditional forms of training. In Britain, generally, change tends to unravel slowly and, while there is something to be said against radical re-constructions, there is also something in Paul Chapman's (1998) remark that were Project 2000 courses to be revamped quickly or radically, 'too much egg would end up on too many well-known faces'.

The most radical change of all would be separate entry for students into their psychiatric programmes with independent control of their curriculum. Although not entirely a homogenous group, a range of factors define psychiatric nursing as different to other branches. Chief among these is the significant number of psychiatric patients who refuse help and who may then be forcibly given medication which they do not want. Psychiatric nurses have, historically, played a key role in how this coercion or 'managing compliance'—to give it its fashionable name—is carried out. This suggests that the nature of psychiatric nursing, as well as the relative position of psychiatric nurses within the State, is markedly different to that of general nurses. Psychiatric nurses are in an ambivalent position because their dual tasks—to be at once therapeutic and custodial—are irreconcilable. Unsurprisingly, there exists quite persuasive, empirically derived data that points to differences in attitude and value systems between general and psychiatric nurses (Clarke, 1989; 1991). Such data tends to be ignored by educationalists, intent on putting idealised notions of what constitutes nursing ahead of what is known about the needs and wants of nurses. In particular, the psychiatric nurse's role in imposing unwanted treatments is left unexplored.

The quantitative-qualitative debate

From the standpoint of practising nurses, debates within 'the academic ascendancy' as to which of these research approaches best suits 'the profession' must seem faintly ludicrous. Irony of ironies, a group of psychiatric nurses already assert the primacy of quantitative approaches (Cannon *et al*, 1999) on the grounds that qualitative research is unscientific and, therefore, of questionable validity.

While a debate such as this might, at first glance, seem esoteric, it encapsulates perfectly the question of whether nursing can be defined in standardised, objective, measurable, evidence-based terms or if, alternatively, it is a personal, narrative based, intuitive, vocational enterprise. This debate has necessarily dwelled on the question of definitions—in nursing the most elusive quest of all. I cannot think of a single definition that has worked: in effect, and harsh though it may sound, there is no such **thing** as nursing, no unifying focus or essence.

And yet the yearning to make nursing acceptably explicit persists. In my view, it would be better to discard notions of definition altogether and ask, instead, which nurses are making which definitions and why. What do definitions achieve for particular sub-groups? How nurse educationalists define nursing care, for instance, may have more to do with their drive for professionalism—traditionally, education has been a gathering point for ambitious nurses—than any dispassionate analysis of what it all might mean. Of course, the educational role hardly stands in the way of having opinions about other groups, and nurse educationalists are quick to wax lyrical on the nature of nursing care, even when, like myself, they haven't seen a patient in years. In fact, an inverse ratio exists where those most involved in patient care are the least likely to pontificate on its nature, whether in journals, conferences, or whatever. One has to look, therefore, at the uses to which particular groups put definitions, and the manner in which language is used to that end. Nurses who deliver care may avoid language that distances them from the practical-scientific concerns of medicine since, by extension, it divorces them occupationally from doctors: there is no evidence that practice-based nurses seek such a divorce, although plenty of evidence that an elite of university-based nurse-lecturers do. Educationalists often behave as if their curricula were out-and-out 'prescriptions for life' and it was in that sense that I took umbrage at the idea of an International Language Classification for Nursing. I had become tired of these 'conceptual frameworks', not just because of their ubiquity, but more so because they reeked of armchair philosophising, bereft of any connection with practice. I concluded, ruefully, that nursing 'frameworks' in general bear most of the hallmarks of a Heath Robinson Machine: terrifyingly impressive at first sight, daunting in its complexity, plausible even, in its practical application. That is, until you ask: 'does it work?'

Truth and validity

The problem with nursing models, classifications, and concepts lies in the difference between truth and validity: making valid conclusions flow from a string of premises can look impressive, but is not all that difficult if you accept the initial premises as being true. However, deriving valid conclusions from arguments does not mean that either their premises (or conclusions) are true. On my desk are six nursing texts, none of which define what nursing is: that is, their initial terms or premises are not related to any concrete referents, but are simply assertions that are then used for the development of elaborate models, logically assembled, internally coherent and semi-plausible, but just not true.

Holden's (1996) work is a good example. Attempting to define nursing knowledge, she utilises what she calls 'non-articulated skills', which she then subsumes within a category of propositional knowledge. Apparently, nurses draw upon propositional knowledge (for example, science), but then marry it to non-articulated perceptual skills in the way of, she says, surgeons. However, and typically, the content of this non-articulated skills base is left unexplained. No effort is made—how could it be?—to explain how something that is 'not articulated' can be understood in propositional terms. Whereas, in the case of surgery, a theory of biological function informs the surgeon's actions, in the case of nursing no such precise, material interventions, informed by theory, are possible. What Holden does is simply link the two—propositions and non-articulation—and, presumably, we are not supposed to see the join.

As I have said, the absence of a sceptical response to such writing results from a certain reluctance to call a spade a spade; perhaps, too, an understandable reticence about attacking a 'profession' whose standing, historically and morally, is high. From a moral perspective, most nurse theorists, however misguided, are well meant; at the very least, they seek to enhance the social standing of nursing. But it is the majority that matter. For most nurses, it hardly makes sense to attempt to transform an essentially unintellectual undertaking into something supposedly cerebral, even highbrow. Ultimately, the highbrow group will have to reconcile themselves to the majority, whose interests may be the same, but who may wish to approach problems from a different perspective. At first sight, it might appear odd to seek to describe, to take one example, the giving of a bed bath at Diploma, Degree and Master's levels! One is forced to ask how patients might **experience** being bathed at Masters as opposed to Diploma level! At the same time, giving someone a bath is not a routine procedure: it is a social encounter rich in possibilities for helping patients. Twigg's (1997) 'deconstructing the social bath' is worth reading in this respect and lends considerable support to the importance of discussing these issues at a variety of levels. Nursing's problems, at this stage of its development, is to imagine that the Master's degree approach is the only way for the profession to move forward. Like medicine and the law, nursing will have to, however reluctantly for some, accommodate itself to different levels of practice. Not everyone can have Master's degrees, or the kinds of intellectual concerns that such degrees support.

Evidence base

A current preoccupation in nursing is to seek 'evidence' that might 'explain' successful nursing interventions. In my opinion, any robust uptake of evidenced-based approaches marks the death of nursing. I say this because nurses, unlike other groups, do not (necessarily) draw upon empirically derived strategies for their interventions, but respond to patients anyway. That is, the nursing imperative is to respond to sick people's needs, even when they have little of curative value to offer; when, in effect, the very idea of an 'evidence base' becomes redundant. I suppose one would see this mainly in the care of the dying, but also, I think, in cases of long-standing psychological illness. There is much to argue about here. For some, (McMahon, 1998) the 'all nursing care' that habitually followed medical failure could be seen as placing nurses in a subsidiary relationship to medicine since it denied them a therapeutic function. Nursing, by definition, is not therapeutic, although it may well function as an adjunct to therapy and facilitate recovery from illness and/or general well-being. This has implications for the training of students. A frequent complaint of post Project 2000 students is that, on entering the educational system, they are drenched in sociological theory, but not shown how to give an injection. What kind of education is it that fails to equip students with the technical requirements of the job? After all, wanting to help is of little avail if one does not know how! And yet, where little of a technical nature is involved, as in care of the dying or in chronic illness, this may be where the purest nursing occurs. Before medicine had discovered its late twentieth century treatments and technology, the scope for nursing was greater than it is today. Anne Rafferty (1996b) has observed that there was a period when the domiciliary nurse could compete with the GP and that the advance of hospitalised medicine acted to bring nurses under medical control. Today, treatments are so efficient that they leave little room for what used to be called 'basic nursing'. In a sense, medical advances have killed 'nursing'. But even if matters were not forced by medical advance, aspiring specialist nurses are simply no longer content to do 'basic nursing' anyway. Probably, most basic nursing now takes place within rehabilitation, hospice, and nursing home settings. As such, we may yet discover what nursing is outside the rarefied echelons of hospital-based consultancy and specialist nursing, recognising that it is about encountering the ordinary miseries of life and relieving misery in a way that is understood by all those involved. The language of everyday life will take care of all of this: international classifications merely deny the inimitable nature of nursing encounters, both at cultural as well as personal levels.

Reflection

Not so, state Brown and Crawford (1999), a formal language is, indeed, needed by the nursing profession. However, apart from recommending 'reflection' as a way of discovering what form this language might take, they say little else. They point out that medical agendas are 'not compatible with nursing philosophies', so that nurses must acquire an 'anti-language' that will (in the patient's interest) compete with the dominant language of medicine. Although they give this language an advocacy function, they remain suspiciously quiet about what its content might be. While appearing to dissociate themselves from Professor Clark's position, they seek a construction wherein nurses take account of 'the power of language' to effect human behaviour. But they are unclear about how nurses would do this, or even of what the nature of this language would be. Part of the problem is their contention that 'we take for granted how we shape the world around us with language'. The alternative view, that language systems are an outcome of culture and hierarchical power systems (such as hospitals, for instance) is just as persuasive (Etzioni, 1960; Gahagan, 1984), as well as being the model that would, probably, fit the experiences of most practitioners.

At least the system espoused by Clark has the advantage of being clean cut, possibly because it is an abstract construction uncluttered by considerations of actual practice. Whereas

Brown *et al* seem not to know what it is that they seek in a nursing language. To further their case, they provide an example of a GP who asks a CPN to 'see this young prostitute with kids who is inadequate and has a personality problem' (Crawford, 1999: p48). According to them, this exchange is an example of 'linguistic entrapment', since the woman turns out, according to the CPN, to be 'well-educated, articulate and with a happily playing child'. My contention is that a common usage (of English) sufficiently deals with this situation; that this is an example of pig-ignorant rudeness on the part of the doctor, and that there is nothing to be gained in redefining it as 'linguistic entrapment' or linguistic anything else.

Nurses speak

Concern over the language that nurses use is important: however, if the moral rules which govern day-to-day relationships are present in nursing, then the language that ordinarily mediates these rules should suffice. What matters in nursing is the belief that patients in treatment settings have not lost their rights to civility and good care, and that the nursing task is to help patients avoid, what Goffman (1961) calls, 'degradation ceremonies' that, in some places, can still occur, particularly during admission procedures.

This is not to say that patients are saints. In their paper, Crawford and Brown (1999) (rightly) describe how nurses, sometimes carelessly, label patients 'devious', 'manipulative', or 'anti-social'. Well, I have nursed a few in my time who were exactly that and, on occasions, it was necessary to say so: in nursing relationships, it cuts both ways. For to assume that patients are not devious or manipulative (when they sometimes obviously are), is to deny to them aspects of common humanity. Finally, I am not so sure that busy surgical wards are the 'richly textured, linguistic environments' that Brown and Crawford (1999) say they are. How often one hears nurses say: 'We don't have time to talk, we are so busy'. To what extent this 'busyness' is a carefully constructed image of selflessness or, alternatively perhaps, a necessary means of avoiding human contact, is difficult to say: but it does suggest an environment where, apart from medical jargon, linguistics takes a low priority.

While debates about the kinds of language that nurses employ might, at first sight, seem esoteric, they encapsulate perfectly questions about the nature of nursing. It might seem strange to outsiders that such a debate could proceed at all in the absence of the definition of basic terms. Yet it does. Eluding every attempt to capture its meaning, nursing has become the Holy Grail of definitions. No wonder that Crawford and Brown admit to 'a huge gap in our knowledge of what nursing language amounts to' and yet they still insist on making it the basis of a 'counter advocacy programme to the practice of medicine within medical settings'.

Conclusion

Both Professor Clark (1999a; 1999b) and Crawford and Brown (1999) are searching for the same thing, but in different ways. Both seek uniformity in a language that will identify nursing and, to some extent, establish nursing's reputation. Professor Clark and her international colleagues have opted for a formulation of magisterial proportions, whereas Crawford and Brown argue from a combative standpoint, where nurses compete with doctors and achieve autonomy by adopting an 'anti-language'.

In her original paper, Professor Clark (1999a) had complained about nurses being saddled with an 'ordinary language' that varied according to context 'and the private understanding of the people using it'. She argued for a standardised language with systematised terms, aggregated and even codified within computer systems. Of course, such systems would benefit managerial decision-making, especially when allocating or auditing resources. In effect, the International Classification Language System is probably not much more than a sophisticated auditing tool, which, like most auditing tools, neglects the distinctive, local elements of nursing encounters.

Brown and Crawford (1999) sought to inflate the importance of contexts to language. In responding to my statements about the uniqueness of nursing encounters, they believed that I had downplayed social factors (such as class differences) in health provision, and they insisted on a political influence on nursing by means of an 'advocacy language'. However, they could not describe the content of this language. In particular, they take exception to my contention that 'the ordinary social and moral rules that govern speech are sufficient for patient care'. This does, perhaps, require revision. These ordinary rules do go a long way towards achieving this end, but are, on reflection, insufficient. Instituting common decency in a treatment setting is sufficient to counteract overt abuses. When the problems of nursing are more subtle, however, something else would seem to be required. The language of assumption, for instance, where older people are deemed incapable of being challenged, can lead to a change of attitude that brings, in its wake, a shift from a dependency to an enabling language. The link with attitude is important. Brown and Crawford (1999), for example, showed how elderly-care nurses sometimes use 'baby talk' with their patients, but branded this an example of 'linguistic abuse'. More a question of cringing condescension perhaps, but, yes, we could do worse than look at the ways in which nurses use language with patients. However, 'enlarging' nursing care, either through international classifications or the imposition of psycho-linguistics, seems to me to be an over-reaching, idealistic activity. Patients need to be treated with civility, honesty, clarity, consistency, respect and, most of all, compassion. In addition, these qualities need to be communicated clearly to them. While these activities do not exhaust the nursing contribution, in many settings they would go a long way towards ensuring good care.

9

The Nurse: Researcher? Ethicist? Professional? Which?

What price research?

*A*t first sight, the relevance of research to nursing seems obvious: it suggests several things. First, that nursing is not just about received ideas, about training, but that it is an educated activity that challenges, and even undermines, traditional practices. It's hard to deny that everybody needs education, and nurses are no different in seeking to test their practice against a body of theory. However, as someone currently involved in the preparation of first level nurses, I am only too aware of how exasperated students are at our failure to provide what they imagine are the skills required to do 'basic nursing care'. What this 'basic nursing care' is, is elusive and it perplexes me that they know what 'it' is, but it seems that they do and that it is more to do with tradition than with academia. Another thing is that this belief in basic nursing care becomes stronger following the student's exposure to practice: perhaps the latter acts to reinforce their beliefs while diminishing whatever faith they might have had in the relevance of theory. What I think happens is that they come to the university—they rarely become of it—already vaguely aware that something is amiss. Their subsequent exposure to psycho-social theorising encourages their suspicion that something really is amiss, and it is at this point that they begin to exclaim 'I came here to be a nurse'. What their visits to clinical placements confirms is their primitive (but correct) intuition that 'the realities' of practice are, indeed, far removed from the sociologese of the classroom. And, of course, the classroom is a lame duck experience; the practice arena being where ultimate sanction lies.

The problem

In my view, the nature of nursing cannot be researched. This is not to devalue what nurses do: on the contrary, it merely says that there is no necessary relationship between explanation and appreciation. One can appreciate from different vantage points the value of nursing, irrespective of whether it is seen as an everyday occurrence; for example, nursing a sick relative, or as a professional enterprise. It is the coexistence of a variety of perspectives that makes nursing difficult to understand. However, of all its different forms, that which most people claim to understand—at an intuitive level—is 'basic nursing care'. It is this concept that, more than any other, bewitches applicants to nursing [most especially general nursing], as well as quickly becoming a stick with which to later beat those who see nursing in more exalted terms. In fact, it is very difficult to define a concept such as basic nursing care. In the first place, either the 'nursing' or the 'care' must be dropped because they are a tautology. We are then left with 'basic nursing', but I think that we can drop the 'basic', too, because, unless we can define 'nursing', trying to define basic nursing is putting the cart before the horse. Researching what cannot be defined is problematic to put it mildly, and it looks as if nurse researchers have, for some years now, been engaged in an underhand practice.

A solution

One group has attempted to solve the research problem by crudely shifting the concerns of nursing so that they resemble the more measurable problems of psychology and medicine. Having done this, they then called for the introduction (to nursing) of research methods more suited to these other disciplines. Hence, the current fixation with randomised controlled trials (RCTs), which, ideally, are best suited to solving problems least likely to have a will of their own; agriculture, for example, where they originated. These RCTs were more fully discussed in *Chapter 5*. Here, I want to draw attention to their influence on definitions of nursing.

Where RCTs are indicated in human problems, the focus of such studies is normally to do with bio-physical-chemical equations, such as double blind drug trials where outcomes can be clinically evaluated. Attempting to utilise RCTs in nursing, where inter-relationships and the experience of illness are the prevailing factors, is another matter. And, indeed, whenever nurse researchers do RCTs, they typically substitute for 'nursing' some other kind of intervention. For example, they might randomly establish groups of people where Group One receives one treatment, as opposed to another group that is given treatment two, and another given no treatment at all. Now, there are huge problems—often glossed over—in constructing these 'random' groups, not the least of which is the issue of consent. For if the sample consists of people with mental illness, then how does the process of consent to treatment work? Little is said about this. In nursing, RCT aficionados, unsurprisingly, often settle for randomising the treatments to be given (rather than the groups) and then looking for results via independent analysis. The question of the random allocation of subjects within these groups, as well as the additional difficulty of their representativeness—given that they have illnesses that are, themselves, ill-defined—become neglected issues. Also, and most importantly, we are now discussing treatments: for example, in a mental health RCT, the treatments might be a comparison between drug therapy, behaviour therapy, or no therapy at all. The nursing element is conveniently sidestepped and understandably so, for if nursing is to do with relationships, then this puts the qualitative cat among the quantitative pigeons. Nursing, to my mind, is just not researchable in this 'scientific' way. Perhaps recognising this, some nurse groups have recoiled from the philosophical problems involved by substituting 'nursing' with 'therapy'. Only an influential minority have followed this course and others have opted for an entirely different way of investigating nursing, namely qualitative research.

Feel the quality

Sufficient accounts of qualitative research exist to prevent me going over this ground again. However, in these studies, the problems are simply reversed. Here, you can analyse and evaluate relationships to your heart's content, except you then have the problem of persuading your audience that what you are doing is actually scientific. Critics of qualitative designs are quick to point out that you cannot generalise from their findings in any acceptable way, nor is it possible—given the nature of these studies—to replicate them: hence, both their validity and reliability are suspect.

Having used both approaches, there are some things to be said both for and against them. First, the deficiencies of qualitative studies are very real, if they are asserted to be scientific: their advantage is that only in this way can internal meanings (of people) be examined and reported. Second, while some might challenge the dependency of quantitative studies on empiricism, such (hypothesis testing) studies are simply the way in which questions to do with physical reality are asked. Having said that, they are inadequate when examining complex human, attitudinal behaviour.

There is no third way, by the way. Attempts to merge irreconcilable approaches to research are both misguided and confusing. One notable attempt at this was Burnard and Hannigan's (2000) call for a synthesis of quantitative and qualitative approaches. This was a classic foray into the land of 'seeing both sides of the story'. Although superficially attractive, such thinking is regressive in a nursing context, with its age-old tendency to defer to more established viewpoints: what Burnard and Hannigan do is put nurses back inside a framework of consensus and accommodation. Clearly, both writers—and they are not alone—are distraught at divisiveness within the profession: plainly, they see disagreement in negative terms. Accordingly, they depict quantitative and qualitative research as a polarisation with separate camps attended by gurus, entrenched, fractious. Although they acknowledge that different kinds of problems require one or other of these approaches, the resultant necessity to retain both avenues seems lost on them. They prefer to work on the premise that qualitative/quantitative debates are about the primacy of one over the other. That some are naively peddling such a view is beside the point: the issue is about the appropriateness of methods in the light of what nursing is. If, for instance, quantitative research were to be sold as some kind of 'gold standard' and not simply as an applicable approach to a given problem, then more than appeasement to such a view is surely required, if, indeed, a case can be made for qualitative research as a valid mode of inquiry. Not to assert the uniqueness of qualitative inquiry is to drain it of vitality and creative edge, to relegate it to the second division. Whether such studies constitute 'science' is not an irrelevant question: at the moment they are the best available approach given that many nursing problems are outside the scope of scientific methods.

Fundable research

Calls for methodological eclecticism are not new (see Avis and Robinson, 1996), but they are, nowadays, hampered by the drive for evidence-based interventions. By evidence is meant 'hard' evidence of the sort that can be communicated graphically, via numbers and flow charts, and which can demonstrate the efficiency of this or that patient intervention. Immediately, we can see that, although there are areas of nursing where this would be possible—areas that involve physical or discrete psychological interventions—there are, equally, areas concerned with human relationships where no such evidence would be forthcoming. Funding is hard to come by for studies concerned with the latter category. If projects do not resemble medical-style research, with their capacity to produce quantitative indices and generalisable results, then they can be seen as unworthy of financial backing or even, in some circles, professional recognition. One unwelcome tendency designed to refute the charges of 'non-scientific' has been for qualitative researchers, whose 'evidence base' is narrative, to couch their work in pseudo-scientific jargon. This, of course, only makes matters worse.

Collaborative research

Others (Ritter 1997) have called for more collaborative approaches, with nurses combining, principally, with medicine in research aimed at problems germane to both professions. This, too, has its pitfalls. Collaboration with the medical profession has, historically, meant accepting their views about matters, and especially implies an acceptance of their methods of inquiry and the playing down of alternative (narrative-based) approaches. Collaboration is likely to be skewed because nothing suggests medical research would accept qualitative approaches as valid. Given the bio-physical nature of their perspective, it could fairly be said, why should they? Of course, this is not what RCT enthusiasts in nursing intend. Their collaboration would involve an unhesitating acceptance of the evidence base of the physical sciences, thus eschewing qualitative work altogether.

Where combinations of qualitative and quantitative approaches do take place, I suspect these result from the tentativeness that attends the application of qualitative principles to nursing problems. Whereas quantitative researchers are typically confident, their qualitative counterparts seem keen to embrace mixed methodologies or, disastrously, to ape quantitative terminology by evolving 'crude analogues' for validity/reliability, such as verifiability, creditability, and so on. This mimicry also makes difficult any defence of 'true' qualitative studies, which, if implemented faithfully, bear little resemblance to scientific research. This is why extravagant scientific claims made on their behalf only detract from the power of their narrative/experiential forms. The ability of these forms to effect change is evident throughout history. Just one example may suffice: 'Sans Everything' (Robb, 1967), a narrative account of the abysmal living standards of hospitalised learning disabilities patients, made more of a difference to patient's lives than fifty quantitative studies. There are many reasons why this type of research is so effective, from the brilliance of the writing (Goffman, 1961), to the sheer accessibility and attractiveness of personal accounts. This touches on an important ethical point, which is that nursing is about making connections with people at a level that they understand. Many of my students tell me that this is what distinguishes nursing from other disciplines; the capacity to make difficult information accessible by patients. It is, therefore, odd that some nurses want to produce scientific studies whose access is restricted, not just in a technical sense, but also in its neglect of the actual views of patients in care.

Research is a commodity

People—chiefly organisations—buy research: research operates within a market place and some practitioners are more adept at 'reading' that market than others. Moreover, some nurses have called on their colleagues to get their act together in this respect, and recognise that doing quantitative research is the only way in which the profession will be taken seriously by government and other funding agencies. The nature of research programmes are, thus, no freer from competitive and politically-driven contexts than any other activity. Opting for particular forms of research, therefore, is partly a product of investigative-realism, a cool appreciation of professional need within given political contexts. But while realism cannot be set aside entirely, there ought to be better reasons for doing research than that it will merit funding. If the kinds of qualitative research that nurses seek to do cannot obtain funding because seen as unorthodox, then this suggests a lack of appreciation of what nursing is. That view is amply demonstrated in the following quote:

> 'Randomised controlled trials are the gold standard for research funders, and the position of nursing at the bottom of the Research Assessment Exercise league table testifies to the very poor standards which characterise most nursing research. This sad position in the league table seems to me to be largely a result of the iconoclastic stance of individuals who claim to represent the nursing research community and who continue to argue the case for fundamentally flawed research methods and for "nursing" as opposed to multidisciplinary research.'
>
> (Gournay, 2000: p622)

Of course, to completely rule out multidisciplinary research would be silly, and nobody seeks to do that. There will always be issues that are of interest to both doctors and nurses, and no doubt other disciplines as well. However, what the 'fundamentally flawed research' jibe fails to recognise is that most nurses are proud of their title and, while the kinds of qualitative research that seems to fit nursing best are, from a scientific perspective, flawed, it is this research that best encompasses the most complex nursing questions. For example, the issue of gender and how it works to influence nursing perspectives has implications for research. Most nurses are women and, while questions of gender have hardly been all the rage, some (Davies, 2000) have cautioned against adopting the top-heavy scientistic veneer that characterises male approaches to the ownership and dissemination of knowledge. At heart, these differences are not just about research methods, but also about the different world views represented by these methods. The quantitative group regard questions about the nature of nursing as an irrelevance: they see philosophies of nursing as essentially second-rate, preferring, instead, to address problems about illnesses and their treatments.

Qualitative nurses, alternatively, seek a heterogeneous approach consistent with the divergent nature of nursing practice, as part of a quest to decipher the protracted question of how nursing is defined. Nurses who dissociate their reputation from medicine will be attracted by different kinds of problems and, equally important, will be in a stronger position to influence affairs from a different vantage point.

A profession should be capable of telling society what it sees as the truth and not in any grand or pompous manner, but by balancing its own requirements against what it sees as an ethical response to the nursing needs of individuals and groups. Some problems, the efficacy of drugs, for example, will require a quantitative research strategy. Where the emphasis is on human experience, then more interactive approaches may be appropriate: here, the necessity for nurses to represent the internal worlds of patients becomes obvious. In addition, where medical research uses people as a means to an end—and there is always something of this in all research—then the nursing response should be to look out for the experimental subject's interests. To that end, it matters that nurses retain the right to choose how to ask questions and it should not matter if their findings are expressed in qualitative form. If nurses articulate the experiences of patients to providers of health care, then they will listen. In a nursing context it is, in any event, the content of what is communicated that matters. To silence nursing, because it refuses to toe the line on what counts as fundable research, or because of a scientistic distaste for argument and dissension, is merely to reinforce nursing as a pretender profession.

A moveable feast

Lastly, it is not surprising that this intensive debate on the qualitative/quantitative question moved from psychology, in the 1950s and 1960s, to nursing in the 1980s and 1990s, the opposing camps within psychiatric nursing becoming especially virulent at times.

The refusal of this debate to 'lie down' is because (like the debate about 'the Euro') it is really about deeper things, about the nature of the profession itself.

Is it a basic profession with a noble past, but essentially concerned with basic things, or is nursing a profession of the old school—learned, elitist and self-governing? Perhaps it can be both. After all, the base activities of legal soliciting (messy divorces and house conveyance procedures) seem to go comfortably hand-in-hand with the grander activities taking place at the bar of the Old Bailey. Why not have basic nursing performed by baseline nurses and leave 'the profession' angle to those who aspire to therapeutic and higher education status. If the latter group agreed to define their new roles separately from basic nursing, then this might help. Given that professionalism is about ascendancy and ownership, it might not be difficult to persuade them to change their identity. But trying to define what nursing is by the research it does is going to be difficult. One could try and circumvent the issues by stating that nursing research is research done by people (still) calling themselves nurses: for instance, one shifts one's focus to doing therapies, which is then researched with randomised control trials. However, while interesting enough in itself, this is not **nursing** research.

The problem lies in the patchwork character of what nursing is: because there is no such **thing** as nursing, no uniqueness in its mix, it becomes very difficult to identify what its research might look like. Of the range of approaches on offer, clearly those that capture the narratives of patients and carers is likely to provide the best fit. Such qualitative studies may not be brain science, and the funders of research may not like them, but they best reflect what it is that basic nursing means. They might equally provide a welcome addition to other types of research, for example, amplifying and refining medical findings in respect of individuals or groups. A nursing research, immersed in the narratives of patients, would undeniably carry authority. Why this does not happen is partly to do with current preoccupations with outcomes and their measurement, partly due to the tricky and difficult-to-define processes that accompany change. It is also due to nursing's lack of reputation as a unified and consistent workforce, its historical deferential relationship to other groups and its practical function as intermediary and 'jack of all trades'.

What is nursing?

The word nursing—like policing or teaching—covers a wide area: it has many implications both overt and covert. Yet, it is surprising how many books and papers are written as if nursing was a unitary concept, as if it denoted a specific set of tasks or concepts. Mackay's (1998) finding that student nurses viewed their new occupation in terms of personal characteristics and not academic achievement suggests that its aspirants perceive nursing as a basic **human** response. The problem, for nurses, is that this may actually be true.

It would be difficult, for instance, to show clear differences between nursing carried out by lay-people, such as patient's relatives, and that performed by professionals. Establishing such a difference on the occupational premise that professionals are paid is problematic, since the question of remuneration is blurred by contemporary calls for payments to be made to informal carers. Perhaps what differentiates lay and professional nursing is that, in addition to getting paid, the latter work to time limits within hospitals. In other words, it is not the nature of nursing that distinguishes the lay from the professional, but the fact of society providing nursing care in cases where families cannot, or will not. In this instance, professional nursing is just nursing by another name. To those who would argue that hospital nurses perform complicated physical interventions, I would reply that these are, by nature, medical interventions, not nursing. Yet differences in the nature of lay and professional nursing remain. For example, attending to strangers involves owning information about them: confidentiality becomes important and, as a result, ethical issues come into play.

Relatives and strangers

Perhaps it is ethics that identifies caring for relatives as opposed to strangers? Are relatives bound by the kinds of ethical codes espoused by professionals? Perhaps. Come to think of it, when they inhabit the role of patients, relatives and strangers have much in common. For instance, their different positions do not impede their common humanity and all that that entails. Does that imply a similar standing in respect of ethical judgements? Probably not. For example, while relatives are not above the law, were they to kill a loved one, a court would likely view this differently to a professional who did the same. Although the same moral strictures apply to both, their different situations will partly determine how their actions are judged. Generally, we assume that compassion for relatives carries more moral weight than its professional counterpart. Indeed, in professional nursing, compassion is nowadays played down in favour of more conceptual constructs like empathy.

What juxtaposing lay and professional nursing does is force the question of whether there can be a defined nursing ethics, or if nurses simply draw upon a general ethics to which they then attach nursing labels. According to philosopher,

Mary Warnock (1998), constructing professional codes merely recasts general ethics so as to make them relevant to this or that profession or organisation.

A distinctive nursing view?

The formulation by nurses of a Code of Conduct (UKCC, 1992) reflected not just growing concern with ethics, but also a determination to claim professional standing. Allmark (1995), for example, notes that educationalists regard 'professionalism' as the most important reason for putting ethics into nursing curricula. Certainly, when occupational groups reach a certain independence threshold, and where they appear conscious of acting from an underlying knowledge base, then they proclaim a Code of Conduct. This, of course, is true for most professional groups and that is fine, except that, like Warnock, I doubt if such codes represent much more than variations in terminology—in keeping with the particular organisations they represent—since the values that underpin them are probably similar. In my view, there cannot be a distinctive medical or nursing ethics and, were we to blend both of these into a kind of health care ethics, I doubt if even this domain would supplant everyday ethics when testing the merits of health care issues. Applying everyday ethics to 'medical' questions might actually be more productive, since both the process and outcome of discussion would not need to be filtered through this or that professional sieve. Dyer (1988) agrees that, in medical ethics, 'familiar moral rules are being applied to particular situations and relationships'. This suggests that a) disagreements about moral codes reflects people's attachment to and participation in different ways of living; and b) that causal connections lie in this direction. In other words, nurses approve of the medical model in mental health because of the standing that this model has in our society; it is not purely an objective, professional choice. Drawing from Moore (1970), Du Toit (1995) uses the phrase **'deformation professionale'** to explain how participation in an occupation—any occupation—can affect one's character and behaviour. Popular stereotypes might be 'the fussy accountant', the 'didactic teacher' or the 'argumentative lawyer'. This is a complex area, but, in general, it seems that participation in events can lead to personal change and that the standards, approved by people, are an idealised extension of that which they participate in. So, in addition to illness, nurses have regard for the morality of their society, but if this regard comes from their way of living then they may need to achieve some consistency between their moral reasoning and the practical requirements of their job. It seems that arguments from relativity carry some force, because variations in moral codes are better explained by observing that they reflect ways of living/working more than they do abstractions about how one ought to live; i.e., occupational 'rules' partly determine one's moral choices—for example, forcing one to rationalise about aspects of patient's problems. Turning this on its head, it might be that professional codes will simply reflect the different issues with which the group has to deal. For example, the difficulties that particular nurses experience (see Pink, 1994), when carrying through injunctions 'to do the patient no harm' [Item One: Code of Professional Conduct (UKCC, 1992)], may involve contradictions, i.e., attempting to maintain professional standards of care in situations of under-funding and poor staffing levels. According to Dyer (1988), self-consciousness about standards of conduct is a defining characteristic of professions, and this is where Codes of Conduct come into their own in judging whether or not individuals conform to the Code. That being the case, these Codes are about the moral reputation of the group and not the integrity of individuals. It follows that group standards may poorly represent individuals and sub-groups within the larger group. Contemporary psychiatric nurses, for instance, might see their values submerged beneath the 'general nursing' concerns of most Project 2000 Programmes (Allen, 1990; McIntegart, 1990). More specifically, a Code may fail to protect individuals who act to uphold it. In the case of Graham Pink, who made a series of complaints about standards of nursing for his elderly patients, the one discernible outcome of his attempt to make the UKCC Code applicable, was the loss of his job.

Although later becoming a member of the UKCC, Pink's views cut little ice with the managers of his hospital, an indication perhaps of the weakness of 'profession' when operating against corporate need. Certainly, the Pink case demonstrates the difficulties in defining practice outside the constraints of custom and practice, as well as the restrictions on care that stem from economics. In psychiatric practice, it was the same story when two nursing students objected to the use of electric treatment (Bailey, 1983): they too were summarily dismissed. Of course, nursing objections to electric treatment are not unusual. However, when they occur they tend to be in the style that Leonard Stein (1978) called the 'doctor nurse game', a type of covert dissent in which the principle of nursing obeisance remains intact. In the case of the two students, it was not their objection to the particular usage of electric treatment that damned them, as much as that they objected to it in principle. This raises the question of what 'autonomous practitioner status' means for nurses.

Stereotypes

Autonomy is a tall order when you have been struggling for years against unfair and somewhat derogatory imagery. Until recently, nurses have coped with a range of stereotypical images, a particularly potent one being, what Kitson (1996) calls, the 'mother-figure' or 'battle axe' with its obvious overtones of good housekeeping and maternal control. In a way, all the professionalising of nursing has been a reaction to this In the past, the participation of nurses in health care seems to have resembled a kind of 'intermediary' (Towell, 1975) at best, or, at worst, 'fellow traveller' (Pilgrim, 1983). In the former, the nurse operates as general factotum, a kind of ward-based almoner: in the latter, he/she voluntarily participates in the medicalisation of people's problems. Other perceptions are Stein's (1978) conspiratorial model, where the nurse acquires a measure of control by covertly 'managing' medical prescriptions. More recently, we have seen the nurse as 'troublemaker', what used to be termed 'whistleblower' (Beardshaw, 1981).

These latter-day concepts hardly match the 'exalted status' perspectives put about by university-based spokespersons for 'the profession'. It is ironic that, having assiduously cultivated a medical role within hospital practice as the primacy means of escaping the Sarah Gamp role (Rafferty, 1996b), some (nurses) now seek to distance themselves from that medical role in the drive for a new reputation as holistic practitioners. At the same time, there are enough studies that point to nurses maintaining their attachment to traditional/institutional styles (Altschul, 1972; Cormack, 1976; Clinton, 1985; Tattam, 1989; Thomas, 1993) not to mention a substantial literature on actual abuse (Martin, 1984; Clough, 1996). It may hardly be surprising, therefore, that the views of practising nurses differ from those whose clinical connections have been severed by their ascendancy into the university system. Whereas the practice nurse is forced to retain a grasp of the practicalities (consequences) of ethical actions, the university-based academic, unencumbered by socio-economic realities, weaves a more visionary agenda.

At this juncture, it might help to look again at whether the lay comparison with professional nursing still stands. It is unlikely that lay nurses—while they would be guided by medical advice—would carry with them general beliefs about the appropriateness of this or that medical view. On the other hand, professional nurses (of all kinds) do have non-medical perspectives on human illness and distress. It is in that sense, therefore, in the sense of fielding a professional viewpoint, that 'the profession' does differ from lay nursing. Of course, the rightness or otherwise of these non-medical views is another matter, as is, also, their utility within medical settings. Within such settings, the medical judgement must, ultimately, prevail in respect of medical matters, and there cannot be much in the life of a patient that does not impinge on his or her illness. However, while this might seem to confer enormous power on physicians, the social situations in which people experience illness lends itself to the kinds of qualitative analysis that nurses can bring to bear on such situations. While not carrying the weight of scientific research, where nurses can show that their concerns stem from a considered analysis of their patient's problems—and includes the patient's viewpoint—then they can reasonably expect to influence decisions and outcome in health care.

Not always the moral high ground

Almost all nursing discussions presuppose a certain moral high ground. If you were to ask the general public to which professional group they would attach moral purpose, the majority would probably say 'nursing'. Indeed, the most common nursing appellations is 'angel'. History, however, does not entirely bear up this concept and there are instances where the standards of care imposed by nurses were poor, either because of slapdash and/or institutionalised thinking, or, even, in some instances, wilfully neglectful. The Audit Commission's Report (2001) into the poor standards of care for elderly patients is ample testimony to this.

Of course, the nature of the job itself can lead to dilemmas of an unresolvable nature. Merely to attempt to nurse people through the problems engendered by their illnesses can lead to more difficulties. For example, a nurse believes in freedom of choice, but may forcibly change a patient's soiled clothes, despite his objections: the nurse does what she does because she has 'illness-driven conception' of what the patient needs. Of course, a nurse may realise that there is a conflict between what she and her patient perceive is actually needed. However, since the nurse has a duty to care for sick people, the conflict is quickly resolved (for most nurses) by over-riding any objections a patient might have.

For Repper and Perkins (1998), very real problems of choice and civil rights exist in questions of this sort. However, these writers quickly resolve the issue, as most do, by suggesting that conscientiousness about civil rights can 'excuse neglect' and, they say, if someone appears dishevelled or dirty, then they are simply not choosing to accept the help at hand. The question of why they are refusing help is left unanswered by the assumption that illness is the determining factor. Since it is illness that has clouded the consciousness of their patients, then it becomes acceptable to provide nursing care, even if it is against the patients will. The duty to care overrides whatever civil liberty 'restrictions' might apply. In fact, most nurses probably do not give much consideration to these ethical difficulties, at least, not in any academic sense. My view would be that, when a nurse over-rides a patient's objections to having his faecal-smelling clothes removed, it is not by appealing to some utilitarian principle—the greatest good of all her patients—that she does this, but from a natural inclination, not dissimilar to a relative's concern. The problems for professional nurses is that the kind of patient behaviour described becomes so familiar that responses to it become mechanical and, occasionally, slip into poor, or even neglectful practice. Such practice is more likely when it is at the beck and call of institutional tradition, so called 'custom and practise'. It is least likely when there is present a measure of self-consciousness about what one's role ought to be. In other words, what becomes important in proclaiming the ethics and professionalism of a distinctive nursing practice is that—irrespective of the truth or otherwise of this—it becomes an instrument by which people are guided towards a better standard of care. In the case of nursing, their collective views about the nature of illness does distinguish them from lay nursing: there cannot be an absolute distinction (from medicine), of course: these matters are about emphasis and the different ways by which nurses interpret illness in conjunction with patients. Nurses might be different in that, to some extent, they provide dual interpretations based on their knowledge **and** the patient's story. That is why they will ask for analgesics for one patient and antidepressants for another with the same condition. A purely medical knowledge might have difficulty comprehending this.

Most institutes of nurse education go too far in proselytising 'unique nursing skills', when those skills are almost always derived from psychology, medicine, or combinations of both. Perhaps a better approach might be to concentrate on elements that equip nurses to work with patients collaboratively and supportively.

However, whether a nursing perspective is possible or whether—in medical settings—it ought to be, remains a difficult question. My hope is that this attempt to deal with it should prove irritating enough to warrant some strong responses.

10
References

Allen C (1990) PK2000 problems. *Nurs Stand* **5**(6): 3–4

Allen D (1996) *The Shape of General Hospital Nursing: The Division of Labour at Work*. Unpublished PhD Thesis. University of Nottingham

Allitt Inquiry (1994) HMSO, London

Allmark P (1995) Can there be a science of caring. *J Medical Ethics* **21**(1): 19–24

Altschul A (1972) *Patient-Nurse Interaction: A Study of Interaction Patterns in Acute Psychiatric Wards*. Churchill Livingstone, Edinburgh

Amis K (1991) *Memoirs*. Penguin Books, Harmondsworth

Asch S (1952) *Social Psychology*. Prentice Hall, Englewood Cliffs, New Jersey

Atkinson P (1999) Health issues that cannot be ignored. *Nurs Times* **95**(50): 18

Audit Commission (2001) *Forget Me Not: Mental Health Services for Older People*. The Audit Commission, London

Avis M, Robinson J (1996) Continuing dilemma in health-care research. *Nurs Times Res* **1**(1): 9–11

Bailey J (1983) ECT or not ECT: that is the question. *Nurs Times* **79**(9): 12–14

Bannister D (1998) The nonsense of effectiveness. *Changes* **16**(3): 218–20

Barker P (1997) Towards a meta theory of psychiatric and mental health nursing. *Mental Health Pract* **1**(4): 18–21

Barker P (2000) Commentaries and reflections on mental health nursing in the UK at the dawn of the new millennium: Commentary 1. *J Mental Health* **9**(6): 617–19

Barker P (2001) Psychiatric caring. *Nursing Times* **97**(10): 39

Barker P, Reynolds W, Stevenson C (1998) The human science basis of psychiatric nursing. *Perspect Psychiatr Care* **34**(1): 5–14

Bauman Z (1989) *Modernity and the Holocaust*. Polity, Cambridge

BBC Television (1989) *The Late Show*. Discussion with Professor Anthony Clare, Thomas Szasz, Professor Ian Kennedy and Clive James, London

Beardshaw V (1981) *Conscientious Objectors at Work: A Case Study,* Social Audit, London

Belknap I (1956) *Human Problems of a State Mental Hospital.* McGraw-Hill, New York

Benner P (1984) *From Novice to Expert: Excellence and Power in Clinical Nursing.* Addison-Wesley, London

Bennett J, Done J, Hunt B (1995) Assessing the side-effects of antipsychotic drugs: a survey of CPN practice. *J Psychiatr Ment Health Nurs* **2**(3): 177–82

Bosanquet N, Gerard K (1985) *Nursing Manpower: Recent Trends and Policy Options: Discussion Paper 9.* Centre for Health Economics, University of York

Boyle M (1990) *Schizophrenia: A Scientific Delusion?* Routledge, London

Bracken P, Thomas P (2001) Evidence-based medicine and advocacy. *Openmind* **107**, January/February: 19

Bradshaw A (1998) Defining competency in nursing, part 2, an analytical review. *J Clin Nurs* **7**(2): 103–11

Brecher B (1998) *Getting What You Want?* Routledge, London

Brechin A, Sidell M (2000) Ways of knowing. In: Gomm R, Davies C, eds. *Using Evidence in Health and Social Care.* Sage Publications, London: 3–25

Brooker C Repper J (1998) *Serious Mental Health Problems in the Community.* Bailliere Tindall, London

Brooker C, White E (1998) *The Fourth Quinquennial National Community Mental Health Nursing Census of England and Wales.* Universities of Manchester and Keele, Keele

Brown B, Crawford P (1999) Putting the debate on nursing language in context. *Nurs Stand* **14**(1): 41–43

Bruni N (1991) Nursing knowledge: processes of production. In: Gray G, Pratt R, eds. *Towards a Discipline of Nursing*: Churchill Livingstone, Edinburgh: 171–90

Buber M (1970) *I and Thou.* T. Clark, Edinburgh

Burnard P (1990) Learning from Experience: Nurse Tutors' and Student Nurses' Perceptions of Experiential Learning. Unpublished PhD Thesis, University of Wales

Burnard P, Hannigan B (2000) Qualitative and quantitative approaches in mental health nursing. *J Psychiatr and Ment Health Nurs* **7**(1): 1–6

Burns T (2000) The legacy of therapeutic community practice in modern community mental health services. *Therapeut Communit* **21**(3): 165–74

References

Caine T, Smail D (1981) *Personal Styles in Neurosis: Implications for Small Group Psychotherapy.* Routledge and Kegan Paul, London

Cannon B, Coulter E, Gamble C *et al* (1999) Personality bashing. *Ment Health Care* **2**(9): 319

Casey A (2001) Language barrier. *Nurs Stand* **15**(18): 24

Chapman P (1998) Degree of scepticism. *Nurs Times* **94**(2): 63

Chinn PL, Kramer MK (1999) *Theory and Nursing: Integrated Knowledge Development,* Fifth edn, Mosby, London

Clare A (1999) Psychiatry's future: psychological medicine or biological psychiatry? *J Ment Health* **8**(2): 109–11

Clark J (1999a) A language for nursing. *Nurs Stand* **13**(3): 422–47

Clark J (1999b) Response from June Clark. *Nurs Stand* **13**(41): 36

Clarke L (1989) The effects of training and social orientation on attitudes towards psychiatric treatments. *J Adv Nurs* **14**(6): 485–93

Clarke L (1991) Attitudes and interests of students and applicants from two branches of the British nursing profession. *J Adv Nurs* **16**(2): 213–23

Clarke L (1996) Participant observation in a secure unit: care, conflict and control. *Nurs Times Res* **1**(6): 431–40

Clarke L (1999a) *Challenging Ideas in Psychiatric Nursing.* Routledge, London

Clarke L (1999b) Spare the rod–protect the child. *Paediatr Nurs* **11**(3): 6–9

Clarke L (1999c) Nursing in search of a science: the rise and rise of the new nurse brutalists. *Ment Health Care* **2**(8): 270–72

Clarke RVG, Cornish DB (1972) *The Controlled Trial in Institutional Research.* HMSO, London

Clay T (1987) *Nurses, Power and Politics.* Heinemann, London

Clinton M (1985) 'Stuck in an educational rut', *Nurs Mirror* **161**, October 23rd: 37–38

Clough R (1996) *The Abuse of Care in Residential Institutions.* Whiting and Birch, London

Cole A (1990) The cosmic crusaders. *Nurs Times* **86**(5): 28–29

Coleman R, Smith M (1997) *Working with Voices: Victim to Victor.* Handsell Press, Runcorn

Coombes R (2001) Same old story about elderly care. *Nurs Times* **97**(14): 12

Cooper D (1961) *Psychiatry and Anti-Psychiatry.* Tavistock Publications, London

Cormack D (1976) *Psychiatric Nursing Observed*. Royal College of Nursing, London

Cormack D (1983) *Psychiatric Nursing Described*. Churchill Livingstone, London

Crawford P (1999) Nursing language: uses and abuses. *Nurs Times* **95**(6): 48–49

Crawford P, Brown B (1999) A language for nursing: furthering the debate. *Nurs Stand* **14**(12): 36–37

Davies C (1998) Caring for health. In: Walmsley J, Northedge A, eds. Block 1, *Who Cares?* K100 Understanding Health and Social Care, The Open University, Milton Keynes: 70–119

Davies C (2000) Care and the transformation of professionalism. In: Davies C, Finlay L, Bullman A, eds. *Changing Practice in Health and Social Care*. Sage, London: 343–54

Department of Health (1998) *Modernising Mental Health Services*. HMSO, London

Department of Health (1999a) *National Service Framework for Mental Health*. Department of Health, London

Department of Health (1999b) *Review of the Mental Health Act 1983: Report of the Expert Committee*. HMSO, London

DHSS (1971) *Report of the Farleigh Hospital Committee of Inquiry*. Cmnd. 4557, HMSO, London

DHSS (1972) *Report of the Committee of Inquiry in Whittingham Hospital*. Cmnd. 4861, HMSO, London

DHSS (1974) *Report of the Committee of Inquiry into South Ockendon Hospital*. HMSO, London

Downe S (1990) A noble vocation. *Nurs Times* **86**(40): 24

Du Toit D (1995) A sociological analysis of the extent and influence of professional socialisation on the development of a nursing identity among nursing students at two universities in Brisbane, Australia. *J Adv Nurs* **21**(1): 164–71

Dyer AR (1988) *Ethics and Psychiatry: Towards a Professional Definition*. American Psychiatric Press Inc., Washington, DC

Edwards G (1992) Does psychotherapy need a soul? In: Dryden W, Feltham C, eds. *Psychotherapy and its Discontents*. Open University Press, London: 194–224

Eisenberg L (1997) Past, present and future of psychiatry: personal reflections. *Can J Psychiatry* **42**(11): 705–13

Elliot H (1997) Holistic nursing and the therapeutic use of self. *Complement Ther Nurs Midwif* **3**(3): 81–82

References

Eraut M (1994) *Developing Professional Knowledge and Competence.* Falmer Press, London

Etzioni (1960) Interpersonal and structural factors in the study of mental hospitals. *Psychiatry* **23**: 13-22

Fanon F (1967) *Black Skin, White Mask.* Grove Press, London

Fawcett J (1993) *Analysis and Evaluation of Nursing Theories.* F A Davis and Company, Philadelphia

Fee D (2000) The broken dialogue: mental illness as discourse and experience. In: Fee D, ed. *Pathology and the Postmodern.* Sage Publications, London: 1–17

Fernando S (1991) *Mental Health, Race and Culture.* Macmillan/Mind, London

Festinger L (1957) *A Theory of Cognitive Dissonance.* Row: Peterson, Evanston: Illinois

Festinger L, Carlsmith JM (1959) Cognitive consequences of forced compliance. *J Abnorm Social Psychol* **58**(8): 203–10

Firby PA (1990) Nursing: a career of yesterday? *J Adv Nurs* **15**(6): 732–7

Fortinash KM, Holoday-Worret P (2000) *Psychiatric Mental Health Nursing.* Mosby, London

Foucault M (1971) *Madness and Civilisation: A History of Insanity in an Age of Reason.* Tavistock, London

Fox N (1993) *Postmodernism, Sociology and Health.* The Open University Press, Buckingham

Frude N (1980) Child abuse as aggression. In: Frude N, ed. *Psychological Approaches to Child Abuse.* Batsford Academic and Educational, London: 136–48

Fulford KWM (1996) Concepts of disease and the meaning of patient-centred care. In: Fulford KWM, Ersser S, Hope T, eds. *Essential Practice in Patient-Centred Care.* Blackwell Science, Oxford: 1–16

Gahagan (1984) *Social Interaction and its Management.* Methuen, London

Garbett R (1996) Second sight. *Nurs Times* **92**(29): 42–43

Gill AA (199) Hunforgiven. *The Sunday Times Magazine* 11th July, 20–23

Godzich W (1984) Forward. In: Chambers R, ed. *Story and Situation: Narrative Seduction and the Power of Fiction.* Manchester University Press, Manchester: xi–xxii

Goffman E (1961) *Asylums.* Penguin Books, Harmondsworth

Glynn I (1999) *An Anatomy of Thought: The Origin and Machinery of the Mind.* Weidenfeld, London

Golden CJ, Sawicki RF (1985) Neurophysiological basis of psychopathological disorders. In: Hartlage LC, Telzrow CF, eds. *The Neurophysiology of Individual Differences*. Plenum Press, London: 203–36

Gostin L (1977) *A Human Condition*. Mind, London

Gournay K (1996) Changes and challenges: the future of mental health nursing. In: Gournay K, Sandford T, eds. *Perspectives in Mental Health Nursing*. Bailliere Tindall, London: 193–95

Gournay K (1998) Face to Face. *Nurs Times* **94**(24): 40–41

Gournay K (2000) Commentaries and reflections on mental health nursihg in the UK at the dawn of the new millennium: Commentary 2. *J Ment Health* **9**(6): 621–23

Gournay K, Brooking J (1994) Community psychiatric nurses in primary health care. *Br J Psychiatry* **165**(8): 231–38

Gournay K, Ritter S (1997) What future for research in mental health nursing. *J Psychiatry Ment Health Nurs* **4**(6): 441–42

Gournay K, Sandford T, Johnson S, Thornicroft G (1997) Dual diagnosis of severe mental health problems and substance abuse/dependence: a major priority for mental health nursing. *J Psychiatr Ment Health Nurs* **4**(2): 89–95

Gray BT (1998a) The politics of psychiatry and community care. *Changes* **16**(1): 24–37

Gray S (1998b) Olanzepine: efficacy in treating the positive and negative symptoms of schizophrenia. *Ment Health Care* **1**(6): 193–94

Gray S, Gournay K (2000) What can we do about extrapyramidal symptoms? *J Psychiatr Ment Health Nurs* **7**(3): 205–11

Halford S (1997) *Gender, Careers and Organisations*. Macmillan, Basingstoke

Handford L (1994) Nursing and the concept of care. In: Hunt G ed. *Ethical Issues in Nursing*. Routledge, London 181–97

Hare R (1963) *Freedom and Reason*. Oxford University Press, Oxford

Hart C (1994) *Behind the Mask: Nurses, Their Unions and Nursing Policy*. Bailliere Tindall, London

Hart C (1999) Swallowing the party line. *Nurs Times* **95**(31): 43

Heath T (1998) Compelling arguments. *Ment Health Care* **2**(1): 10–11

Heider F (1958) *The Psychology of Interpersonal Relations*. Wiley, New York

Hicks C (1998) The randomised control trial: a critique. *Nurse Researcher* **6**(1): 19–32

References

Higgs R (1996) Comment on Chapter 1. In: Fulford, KWM, Ersser S, Hope T eds. *Essential Practice in Patient-Centred Care.* Blackwell Science, Oxford: 17–21

Holden RJ (1996) Nursing knowledge: the problem of the criterion. In: Kikuchi JF, Simmons H, Romyn D, eds. *Truth in Nursing Inquiry.* Sage, London: 19–35

Howitt D (1998) *Crime, the Media and the Law.* John Wiley and Sons, Chichester

Humphreys J (1996) English nurse education and the reform of the health service. *J Educ Policy* **11**(6): 655–59

Jackson C (1999) Horses for courses. *Ment Health Learn Disabil Care* **2**(12): 410–11

Johnston P (1998) Nursing crisis blamed on cultural failure. *The Daily Telegraph,* October 26th: 7

Jones K (1972) *A History of the Mental Health Services.* Routledge & Kegan Paul, London

Jones M (1982) *The Process of Change.* Routledge, London

Jones M (1952) *Social Psychiatry.* Penguin Books, Harmondsworth

Kee R (1980) *Ireland: a History.* Weidenfeld & Nicolson, London

Keen T (1999) Schizophrenia: orthodoxy and heresies. a review of alternative possibilities. *J Psychiatr Ment Health Nurs* **6**(6): 415–24

Keighley T (2001) At the heart of nursing. *Nurs Stand* **15**(16): 24–25

Keltner N (1996) Psychoanatomy of schizophrenia. *Perspect Psychiatr Care* **32**(2): 32–35

Kitson A (1993) *Nursing: Art and Science.* Chapman & Hall, London

Kitson A (1996) Does nursing have a future? *Br Med J* **313**(7022): 1647–51

Kitwood T (1988) the contribution of psychology to the understanding of senile dementia. In: Gearing B, Johnson M, Heller T, eds. *Mental Health Problems in Old Age.* John Wiley & Sons, Chichester: 123–30

Kohn M (1999) *As We Know It: Coming to Terms with an Evolved Mind.* Granta, London

Kuhn T (1970) *The Structure of Scientific Revolutions.* University of Chicago Press, Chicago

Lambert MJ (1992) Psychotherapy outcomes research: implications for integrative and eclectic therapists. In: Norcross JC, Goldfried MR, eds. *Handbook of Psychotherapy Integration.* Basic Books, New York: 94–129

Lang B (1990) *Act and Idea in the Nazi Genocide.* Chicago University Press, Chicago

Le Var R (1997a) Project 2000: a new preparation for practise—has policy been realised? Part 1. *Nurse Educ Today* **17**(3): 171–77

Le Var R (1997b) Project 2000: a new preparation for practice—has policy been realised? Part 2. *Nurse Educ Today* **17**(4): 263–73

Laing RD (1961) *The Divided Self*. Penguin Books, Harmondsworth

Lipley N (2000) Prescription for change. *Nurs Stand* **14**(27): 11–12

London Observer (2000) Suicide gene found. January 30th:4

Mackay L (1998) Nursing: will the idea of vocation survive? In: Abbott P, Meerabeau L, eds. *The Sociology of the Caring Professions*. 2nd edn. UCL Press, London: 54–72

MacLeod Clark J, Maben J, Jones K (1996) *Project 2000: Perceptions of the Philosophy and Practice of Nursing*. English National Board for Nursing, London

Mair M (1989) Recent rhetoric in he NHS: the language of marketed care. *Asylum* **4**(1): 31–35

Marrin M (1999) Nurses are the problem. *The Sunday Telegraph,* January 10th: 31

Martin JP (1984) *Hospitals in Trouble*. Blackwell, Oxford

Martin E (1999a) *Nurses and Higher Education*. Council of Deans and Heads of UK University Faculties, London

Martin E (1999b) Switched on. *Nurs Times* **95**(12): 52–53

Maslow A (1987) *Motivation and Personality*. Harper & Row, London

Mathieson A (2000) Did nurses aid the Nazis? *Nurs Times* **96**(48): 26–27

May T (1993) The nurse under physician authority. *J Medical Ethics* **19**(4): 223–27

McIntegart J (1990) A dying breed. *Nurs Times* **86**(39): 71

McMahon R (1998) Therapeutic nursing: theory, issues and practice. In: McMahon R, ed. *Nursing as a Therapy*. Stanley Thornes Publishers, Cheltenham: 1–25

Mental Health Nursing Review Team (1994) HMSO, London

Mental Health Syllabus (1982) English National Board for Nursing and Midwifery, London

Meerabeau L (1998) Project 2000 and the nature of nursing knowledge. In: Abbott P, Meerabeau L, eds. *The Sociology of the Caring Professions*. UCL Press, London: 82–105

Menzies I (1960) *The Functioning of Social Systems as a Defence Against Anxiety*. Centre for Applied Social Research, Tavistock Institute, London

Menzies-Lyth I (1988) *Containing Anxiety in Institutions.* Free Association Books, London

Midgley M (2001) *Science and Poetry.* Routledge, London

Milgram S. (1974) *Obedience to Authority: An Experimental View.* Tavistock Publications, London

Minders (1995) BBC Television, April 24th

Moore WE (1970) *The Professions: Roles and Rules.* Russell Sage, New York

Morrall P (1998) *Mental Health Nursing and Social Control.* Whurr, London

Mullen P (1983) *Working with Morality.* Edward Arnold, London

Munro R (1999) Plan to slim down P2000's core. *Nurs Times* **95**(30): 5

Munro R (2001) Ghost of gay 'sickness' haunts nursing. *Nurs Times* **97**(5): 10–11

Murray I (1999) Back to the bedpans for student nurses. *The Times* January 16th: Front Page

National Schizophrenia Fellowship (1999) *Better Act Now!* NCF, London

Nesse RM, Williams GC (1995) *Evolution and Healing: The New Science of Darwinian Medicine.* Weidenfeld & Nicolson, London

Newman MA (1993) *Health as Expanding Consciousness.* CV Mosby, St. Louis

NHS Direct (1997) *The New NHS: Modern, Dependable.* The Stationary Office, London

Nursing Times (1999a) Murders by disordered offenders half 1979 rate **95**(2): 10

Nursing Times (1999b) New brooms remove stain of abuse. **95**(13): 6

Nursing Times (1999c) Nursing is a vocation. **95**(25): 33

O'Reilly J (1999) University in £8m crisis faces break up. *The Sunday Times* February 21st: 5

Paley G, Shapiro D (2001) Evidence-based psychological interventions in mental health nursing. *Nurs Times* **97**(3): 34–5

Perrin S, Spencer C (1981) Independence or conformity in the Asch experiment as a reflection of cultural and situational factors. *British Journal of Social Psychology* **20**(4): 205–9

Phillips M (1999) How the college girls destroyed nursing. *The Sunday Times* January 10th: 13

Pilgrim D (1983) Politics, psychology and psychiatry. In: Pilgrim D, ed. *Psychology and Psychotherapy: Current Trends and Issues.* Routledge and Kegan Paul, Henley: 121–38

Pink G (1994) Heads in the sand. *Nurs Stand* 8(44): 48–49

Plato (1955: Penguin Edition) *The Republic*. Penguin Books, Harmondsworth

Popper K (1959) *The Logic of Scientific Discovery*. Hutchinson, London

Raatikainen R (1997) Nursing care as a calling. *J Adv Nurs* 25(6): 1111–15

Rafferty AM (1996a) *Nursing History and the Politics of Welfare*. Routledge, London

Rafferty AM (1996b) *The Politics of Nursing Knowledge*. Routledge, London

Ramcharan P (1998) *Residents Rights for People with Learning Disabilities Living in Large Hospitals*. Bangor Centre for Social Policy, Research and Development, Summer: 5–8

Redfern L (2000) Watch out, this is going to be big. *Nurs Times* 96(17): 21

Repper J (2000) Adjusting the focus of mental health nursing: incorporating service users' experiences of recovery. *J Ment Health* 9(6): 575–87

Repper J, Perkins R (1998) A tricky act to follow. *Nurs Times* 94(11): 36–37

Ritter S (1997) Taking stock of psychiatric nursing. In: Tilley S, ed. *The Mental Health Nurse: Views of Practice and Education*. Blackwell Science, Oxford: 94–117

Rivett G (1998) *From Cradle to Grave: Fifty Years of the NHS*. King's Fund, London

Robb B (1967) *Sans Everything: A Case to Answer*. Nelson, London

Robbins Committee on Higher Education. (1963) Cmnd. 2154, HMSO, London

Robinson J (1991) Project 2000: the role of resistance in the process of professional growth. *J Adv Nurs* 16(7): 820–24

Rapoport R (1960) *The Hospital as Community*. Tavistock, London

Rogers C (1951) *Client Centred Therapy: Its Current Practice, Implications and Theory*. Constable, London

Rogers C (1978) *Carl Rogers on Personal Power*. Constable, London

Rose S (1998) Brains, minds and the world. In: Rose S, ed. *From Brains to Consciousness?* Allen Lane, London: 1–17

Salvage J (1985) *The Politics of Nursing*. Heinemann, London

Sargant W (1967) *The Unquiet Mind*. Heinemann, London

Scott PA (1998) *Authority and Nursing Knowledge*. Nursing Philosophy Conference, University of Wales, Cardiff, September 12th

Scull A (1996) Asylums: utopias and realities. In: Tomlinson D, Carrier J, eds. *Asylum in the Community*. Routledge, London: 1–6

Scruton R (1995) *A Short History of Modern Philosophy: From Descartes to Wittgenstein.* Routledge, London

Shoenberg E (1980) Therapeutic communities: the ideal, the real and the possible. In: Jansen E, ed. *The Therapeutic Community.* Croom Helm, London: 64–71

Smith P, Agard E (2000) Care costs: towards a critical understanding of care. In: Davies C, Finlay L, Bullman A, eds. *Changing Practice in Health and Social Care.* Sage, London: 211–20

Sontag S (1983) *Illness as Metaphor.* Penguin Books, Harmondsworth

Stanley N, Manthorpe J, Penhale B (1999) *Institutional Abuse: Perspectives Across the Life Course.* Routledge, London

Stein L (1978) The doctor-nurse game. In: Dingwall R. McIntosh J, eds. *Readings in the Sociology of Nursing.* Churchill Livingstone, Edinburgh: 107–17

Tattam A. (1989) Blowing the whistle. *Nurs Times* **85**(23): 20

Thomas A (1993) No room for change. *Nurs Times* **89**(16): 34–36

Tilley S (1998) *Sustaining Varieties of Practice.* Paper presented at The ENB National Mental Health Conference, Robinson College, Cambridge: 29–30 June

Tilley S, Ryan D (2000) Reviewing the literature constricting the field: accounting for the CPN in practice and research. *J Ment Health* **9**(6): 589–604

Towell S (1975) *Understanding Psychiatric Nursing,* Royal College of Nursing, London

Tschudin V (1999) *Nurses Matter: Reclaiming our Personal Identity.* Macmillan, London

Turgenev I (1965) *Fathers and Sons.* Penguin Books, Harmondsworth

Twigg J (1997) Deconstructing the social bath: help with bathing at home for older and disabled people. *J Social Policy* **26**(2): 211–32

UKCC (1992) *Code of Professional Conduct for the Nurse, Midwife and Health Visitor 3rd ed.* HMSO, London

Walden G (1996) *We Should Know Better: Solving the Educational Crisis.* Fourth Estate, London

Wallace C (1987) *For Richer, For Poorer: Growing Up In and Out of Work.* Tavistock, London

Wardwaugh J, Wilding P (1998) Towards an explanation of the corruption of care. In: Allott M, Robb M, eds. *Understanding Health and Social Care: An Introductory Reader.* Sage London: 212–29

Warnock M (1998) *The Intelligent Person's Guide to Ethics*. Duckworth, London

Warren J, Harris M (1998) Extinguishing the lamp: the crises in nursing. In: Anderson CD, ed. *Come Back Miss Nightingale: Trends in Professional Training*. The Social Affairs Unit, London: 11–35

Watson J (2000) Seminar at the University of Brighton. September 22nd, at Falmer

White E (1998) Ethical dilemmas: a solution for community nursing. *Commun Practit* **71**(3): 100–102

White R (1986) *Political Issues in Nursing Vol. 2*. John Wiley, Chichester

Williamson J (1998) Nursing grudges. *The Daily Telegraph* March 1st :32

Witz A (1994) The challenge of nursing. In: Gabe J, Kelleher D, Williams G eds. *Challenging Medicine*. Routledge, London: 23–35

Wray SJ (1994) Schizophrenic sufferers and their carers: a survey of understanding of the condition and its treatment, and of satisfaction with services. *J Psychiatr Ment Health Nurs* **1**(2): 115–23

Index